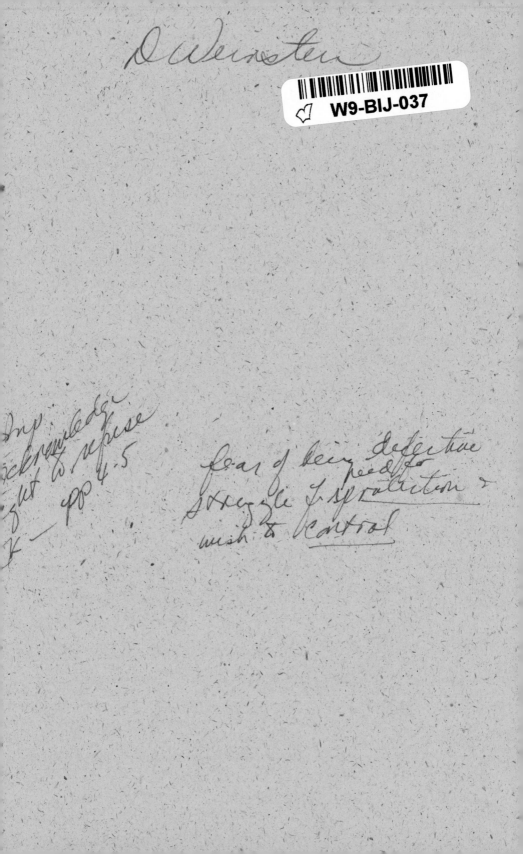

D Weinstein

Imp:
acknowledge
right to refuse
X — pp 4.5

fear of being defective
struggle for gratification &
wish to control

Therapies for Adolescents

Current Treatments for Problem Behaviors

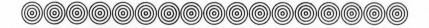

Michael D. Stein
J. Kent Davis

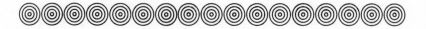

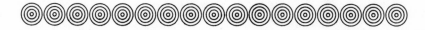

Therapies
for Adolescents

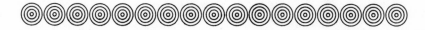

Jossey-Bass Publishers
San Francisco • Washington • London • 1985

THERAPIES FOR ADOLESCENTS
Current Treatments for Problem Behaviors
by Michael D. Stein and J. Kent Davis

Copyright © 1982 by: Jossey-Bass Inc., Publishers
433 California Street
San Francisco, California 94104
&
Jossey-Bass Limited
28 Banner Street
London EC1Y 8QE

Library of Congress Cataloging in Publication Data
Main entry under title:

Therapies for adolescents.

(Guidebooks for therapeutic use)
Includes bibliographies and index.
1. Adolescent psychotherapy. 2. Adolescent
psychopathology. I. Stein, Michael D.
II. Davis, J. Kent. III. Series.
RJ503.T44   616.89'14   81-20761
ISBN 0-87589-513-1   AACR2

Manufactured in the United States of America

JACKET DESIGN BY WILLI BAUM

FIRST EDITION
First printing: February 1982
Second printing: January 1983
Third printing: April 1985

Code 8204

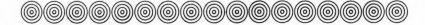

The Jossey-Bass
Social and Behavioral Science Series

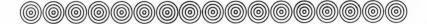

GUIDEBOOKS FOR THERAPEUTIC PRACTICE
Charles E. Schaefer and Howard L. Millman
Consulting Editors

Therapies for Children: A Handbook of Effective
Treatments for Problem Behaviors
Charles E. Schaefer and Howard L. Millman
1977

Therapies for Psychosomatic Disorders in Children
Charles E. Schaefer, Howard L. Millman,
and Gary F. Levine
1979

Therapies for School Behavior Problems
Howard L. Millman, Charles E. Schaefer,
and Jeffrey J. Cohen
1980

*Therapies for Adolescents: Current Treatments
for Problem Behaviors*
Michael D. Stein and J. Kent Davis
1982

**Group Therapies for Children and Youth:
Principles and Practices of Group Treatment**
Charles E. Schaefer, Lynnette Johnson,
and Jeffrey N. Wherry
1982

*Therapies for Adults:
Depressive, Anxiety, and Personality Disorders*
Howard L. Millman, Jack F. Huber,
and Dean R. Diggins
1982

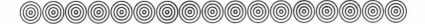

Preface

There are a variety of psychological problems that commonly occur during the adolescent period. This book surveys new developments in techniques of therapy that have proven useful in preventive and ameliorative treatment. It is intended to serve as a reference source for those directly involved in therapeutic work with adolescents and their families.

Recent years have witnessed an enormous expansion in literature on methods of treatment for all age groups. Behavior therapy approaches, especially, have been applied to increasing numbers of problems and patient groups; and the term now encompasses numerous distinct approaches such as operant reinforcement, desensitization, covert sensitization, implosive therapy, and cognitive therapy. Literature in the field of family therapy is also proliferating.

Many articles have appeared that describe the application of new treatment techniques to specific problems. Previous volumes in this series, including *Therapies for Children, Therapies for Psychosomatic Disorders in Children,* and *Therapies for School Behavior Problems* have all proven useful in making this literature accessible to the practicing clinician. The authors are confident that a survey of procedures applicable to the special problems of adolescents will also fill an unmet need.

Overview: Our general approach stems from a recognition of the therapeutic advantage of treatment plans that build upon the variety of techniques effective in treating a given problem. We believe that careful integration of psychodynamic and family therapy orientations with behavior therapy techniques greatly enhances therapeutic effectiveness.

This book follows the digest format that has been so successful in the previous three books. We have condensed more than a hundred articles by eliminating technical research data and highlighting that which is clinically relevant. (Permission to digest articles was given by individual authors, and where such permission could not be obtained, only a brief summary is presented under Additional Readings). This puts immediately into the hands of clinicians data regarding the range of treatment strategies applicable to particular problems and the probable effects of those interventions.

The majority of articles are behaviorally oriented. This is so for two reasons. First, there is more current activity in the theoretical and methodological development of behavioral psychology than in that of more traditional approaches; and secondly, since treatment approaches based on learning theory stress specific interventions for specific problems, a great deal of literature in this area is directly applicable to the purposes of this book.

It would nevertheless be a disservice for us to overlook important contributions to the field of adolescent therapy made by therapists representing other viewpoints. In particular, the literature on dynamically oriented psychotherapy contains much useful information on the therapist-patient relationship, and we have included such articles whenever applications to specific problems are demonstrated. While recognizing the importance of relationship, we wish to emphasize that effective treatment involves much more than the working through of relationship difficulties between therapist and patient.

The chapter headings and subheadings in this volume are intended to assist the clinician in using a problem-oriented approach to developing a treatment plan. As available literature permitted, we have kept these consistent with the current edition of the Diagnostic and Statistical Manual of the American Psychiatric Association (DSM-III) so that once a diagnosis has been made, the clinician will have at his or her fingertips a variety of approaches that have already proven effective in the treatment of that problem.

It should be noted that we have in no way attempted to provide a critical review of the research bases for the techniques presented. Rather we have concentrated on providing a detailed description of interventions and outcomes. The reader is urged to consult original sources and to form his own opinions about theoretical implications. Students and new clinicians, especially, should use this book as a guide to treatment strategies while at the same time reviewing original research and consulting manuals describing specific approaches to therapy.

We wish to thank all those who have contributed to this work: the authors who graciously consented to having digests of their articles included; our professional colleagues, who have stimulated our thinking and helped us to refine our ideas; Lorna McDonald, Carmel Fedors, and Lynn Sabol, who provided expert library assistance; Cecile Stein and Mildred Perkins, who assisted in the typing of the manuscript; and finally, our families, who put up with us and supported us through a long, time-consuming project.

February 1981   Michael D. Stein
                                                                    White Plains, New York

                                                                             J. Kent Davis
                                                            Hastings-on-Hudson, New York

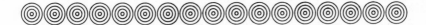

Contents

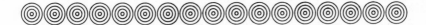

Chapter 2: Physical Disorders   63

    L. R. Pendleton, J. L. Shelton, and S. E. Wilson
Treating Social Anxiety by Desensitization—
    H. Arkowitz
Additional Readings

Chapter 4: Antisocial Behavior   187

Running Away   190

    Classifying Runaways and Selecting Treatment—
        J. D. Orten and S. K. Soll
    Treating Runaway Adolescents with Overinvolved
        Parents—*G. L. Cary*
    Psychotherapeutic Beginnings for Impulsive
        Adolescents—*J. Weinreb and R. M. Counts*
    Additional Readings

Fire Setting   199

    Family and Individual Treatment—*G. A. Awad and
        S. I. Harrison*
    Fire Fetish Treatment by Multiple Behavioral
        Procedures—*S. D. Lande*
    Additional Readings

Aggressive Behavior   206

    A Social Skills Approach to Aggression—*J. P. Elder,
        B. A. Edelstein, and M. M. Narick*
    Reducing Assaultive Behavior by a Self-Control
        Procedure—*S. I. Pfeiffer*
    Additional Reading

Acting Out   212

    A Psychoanalytic Approach to the Acting-Out
        Adolescent—*J. F. Masterson*
    A Multiple Approach Stressing Individual Therapy
        and External Controls—*J. Chwast*
    Use of Rational Behavior Therapy—
        M. C. Maultsby, Jr.

Contents

Chapter 5: Sexual Problems   265

The Authors

Michael D. Stein is currently Chief Psychologist in the Psychiatry Department at Elmhurst Hospital in New York. Prior to this, he was Director of Psychology at Hall-Brooke Hospital, a private psychiatric facility serving adolescents and adults in Westport, Connecticut. He is also in private practice with the Psychological and Educational Services of Westchester. He received the Ph.D. in clinical psychology in 1974 from the City University of New York, after completing an internship at Montefiore Hospital and Medical Center in New York. For about five years he was a supervising psychologist at the Children's Village, a residential treatment center in Dobbs Ferry, New York, which serves children and adolescents. During most of that time he directed the Village's APA-approved clinical psychology internship training program. He also provided clinical and consultative services to the Group Homes and Foster Care and Adoption Units. His interest in innovative therapies for adolescents was augmented by his experiences as therapist for residents who had been notably resistant to therapy for years.

In addition to working with treatment services, he maintains an interest in group and organizational processes and has been a staff member of several group relations training conferences. Other professional affiliations include the International Neuropsychological Society, the Division of Clinical Psychology of the American Psychological Association, and the Westchester County Psychological Association. He has taught psychology at the City College of New York and Lehman College.

Michael Stein lives in White Plains, New York, with his wife Cecile, a speech and language pathologist, and their sons Peter and Nathanael.

J. Kent Davis is Assistant Professor and Chief of Psychological Services for the Department of Pediatrics of the New York Medical College. He received his Ph.D. in psychology from Syracuse University and completed a clinical psychology internship at the Astor Home for Children in Rhinebeck, New York. Prior to coming to the New York Medical College, he served as Supervising Psychologist and Research Coordinator at the Children's Village, a residential treatment center for emotionally disturbed children located in Dobbs Ferry, New York. His work at the medical college involves the education and training of pediatricians in the prevention, early detection, and management of psychological problems in their pediatric patients. He is Behavioral Science Coordinator for a large-scale, federally funded program to train pediatricians as primary health care providers.

Kent Davis maintains a private practice providing therapy for children and adolescents and has special interest in those with learning disabilities and with psychological complications associated with physical illness and disability. He has written and lectured on the evaluation of therapy and special education programs and has developed a comprehensive behavioral science curriculum for pediatricians. He is a member of the American

Psychological Association, the Westchester County Psychological Association, and the Association for the Advancement of Psychology. Kent Davis resides with his wife and children in Hastings-on-Hudson, New York.

Therapies for Adolescents

Current Treatments for Problem Behaviors

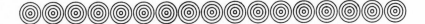

Introduction

The period of adolescence is marked by uncertainty of onset and unclear duration. The claim has been made that it is beginning at younger ages, both physiologically and culturally. At the other end, the term "delayed adolescence" is used to describe a person whose behavior suggests that important developmental tasks commonly ascribed to this period have not yet been completed. This book is concerned with the range of effective therapeutic responses to the special problems of the adolescent. The techniques described have two targets—to assist the adolescent with the developmental tasks and to provide assistance with the behavior problems that signal the adolescent is having difficulty with these tasks.

One of these tasks is coming to terms with physical

1

changes. The need for mastery over one's body, with implications of increased strength and developing sexual characteristics
and reproductive capacities, suggests a variety of potential problems. For both boys and girls, physical development can be a
source of competition, envy, frustration, and feelings of pride
or deep inadequacy. Many factors hamper adjustment to this
new situation. There is, for example, the process of continual
physical change, so that individual triumphs or frustrations
may be of uncertain duration. For a young person with a limited time perspective, the instability of this period can be unsettling.

A further complicating factor is that at the point of early
adolescence, only childhood cognitive strengths and behaviors
are available. When peer pressures, body changes, and related
problems of the early teens commence, the youngster may well
feel excitement mixed with distress, confusion, and other emotions in this important changing situation. The experience of
new possibilities and lack of practice and familiarity in managing them is keenly felt. The need for development of capabili-
ties in so many arenas at once is particularly stressful. The adolescent tends to see behavioral choices in terms of black and
white and to lack the cognitive maturity for coping effectively
with all this complexity.

Certain behaviors are observed to be typical of the early
adolescent period. The intimate secrecy and preoccupation
with sexual implications, the contrasting tomboy and feminine
activities of young adolescent girls, and increased activity levels
and aggressiveness predominantly seen in boys are just some of
the patterns observers note as marking the beginning of the new
stage (see P. Blos, *On Adolescence,* New York: Free Press,
1962). Of great importance also are the loosening and modification of ties to parents and authority figures and sharp changes
in ways of relating to peers. There is ambivalence about relations with the opposite sex. Peer group opinion is a particularly
powerful influence. Adolescents have a paucity of methods and
successful responses to these situations.

Adolescents' attempts to assert independence through rebellious behavior are a matter of common observation. Less

clearly noted, but still of major importance, are the continuing needs for security and closeness, which the youngster still values, but also rejects as childish. This conflict is a major obstacle to the teenager's acceptance of help.

Issues in Beginning Treatment

The adolescent's conflicting feelings about accepting closeness and security also clearly hinders accepting advice and direction. This is one of several issues the clinician must consider when choosing a therapeutic approach. A related issue is how the need for help is presented to the young client. This can decidedly affect the adolescent's willingness to accept both the general idea of seeing a therapist and any specific recommendations for treatment of specific symptom behaviors. Problems can be alleviated through discussion beforehand between the therapist and parents as to how to present the reasons for seeing the therapist. This is particularly true for the younger adolescent.

Several authors have pointed out the differences in treating early versus middle or late adolescents (see Blos, 1962, and M. Harley, "On Some Problems of Technique in the Analysis of Early Adolescents," *Psychoanalytic Study of the Child,* 1970, 25, 99-121, for an extended discussion of these differences). The manner of the child's entry into the treatment relationship is influenced by the stage of the adolescent process at which the child is functioning. Harley, for example, refers to observations by Helene Deutsch that in the beginning work with young adolescent girls, the figure of the doctor evokes major difficulties in communication, as girls of this age are often having difficulty in their relationships with their mothers, and the doctor figure and the mother figure may initially be blurred. Deutsch advised taking the role of the confidante or chum as the best approach to such clients.

Some adolescents clearly indicate that they are actively opposed to seeing a therapist. This may be so for several reasons. One is the child's conclusion that because his parents want him to see a therapist, he must be crazy, a "psycho," or something similarly negative. The assumption is that he is basically defective, and the fact of recommendation to a therapist means that his defectiveness, which heretofore may have been an object of private concern, is about to become public. Harley indicates that the expression of this fear at the beginning of contact between child and therapist is an important issue that must be handled effectively if a treatment alliance is to be established. She recommends that the client be assisted in acknowledging and exploring this fear so that it does not become a stumbling block in the relationship.

Young patients at the first meeting commonly say there is nothing wrong and no good reason for this meeting. At times the presenting problems are the subject of much struggle between teenager and parents, and the admission of difficulties is seen as surrender. This minimizing of one's problems is then extended to the doctor's office. The young client's assumption is that the therapist will try to achieve the parents' goal by the same means. The response to the therapist is an attempt to frustrate what may be perceived as attempts to control or influence him in familiar patterns.

Issues Surrounding the Therapeutic Relationship

It is a point of common agreement in writings on technique with adolescents that the therapist should not attempt to influence the patient in ways the parents have tried (clearly without the desired success). The problem is to make an effective therapeutic contact, recognizing the importance of the control issue and the meaning of the adolescent's denial of problems. The adolescent may begin the first session with the conviction that he and the clinician are on opposite sides of the struggle. The goal is to move toward possible cooperative efforts.

In her writing on dealing with adolescent resistance to therapeutic help, Rogers recommends the acknowledgment of the right to refuse treatment (R. Rogers, "The 'Unmotivated' Adolescent Who Wants Psychotherapy," *American Journal of Psychotherapy,* 1970, *24,* 411-418). She describes several instances from twenty-three clients who were seen who rejected treatment. Subsequently, all returned for help. She illustrates that the right to refuse treatment implies that the option to choose belongs to the young client. This may in some cases be a necessary step in placing the burden of responsibility for problems and their successful solution upon the defiant client.

Werkman points out that differences in values, experiences, and outlook are additional aspects of the gap between adolescent and therapist (S. L. Werkman, "Value Confrontations Between the Therapists and their Adolescent Patients," *American Journal of Orthopsychiatry*, 1974, *44*, 337-344). It is helpful, he argues, for the therapist to be aware of current waves of interests of adolescents, such as in musical groups, self-help fads, and slang. Demonstrating that one is at least partially cognizant of these is a basis for raising the issue of value differences and whether the therapist's goal is to undermine these beliefs and values. Discussion relating to personal fears regarding relationships can follow naturally.

The patient's expectations concerning the role the therapist is expected to play are also important. The common expectation is that the professional is a "hired gun," charged with converting the patient's thinking by invalidating or belittling his convictions or conclusions. A patient who arrives at the office with these assumptions is probably prepared to resist influence. Techniques such as those Rogers outlines provide an early sign of the therapist's independence from parental influence and can lead to discussion of therapist and patient responsibilities.

The therapist can use the reality that he or she is an adult who has already passed through this and subsequent stages. The patient may not believe that the therapist can see across the generation gap. The therapist can share, in an appropriate and timely fashion, his or her own experience of the struggles that the client is currently undergoing. Josselyn describes the discussion at a timely moment of a patient's discovery of her being married and a mother, as well as a professional (I. M. Josselyn, "Psychotherapy of Adolescents at the Level of Private Practice," in B. H. Balser (Ed.), *Psychotherapy of the Adolescent,* New York: International Universities Press, 1957). This information had a major impact on the youngster's struggle to see herself as having a variety of possible simultaneous goals in life.

Harley (1970) describes what she sees as two major issues early in treatment. One is the fear of being defective, previously discussed. The other is the struggle within the adolescent between the wish for control and the desire to be protected. The adolescent rarely perceives this as an internal problem, but rather as the battle between one's own desires for independence and autonomy versus the externally imposed control or repressive efforts of parents and authorities. The role of controlling agent is easily distorted; the intents or the meanings of parental acts can be mistaken and misperceived. The new adolescent patient may therefore expect that the therapist's main objective is toward suppression of independence. The therapist needs to help the patient see the struggle as at least partly one of his or her own inner conflicts.

The problem of beginning a treatment relationship is more difficult with the adolescent who is heavily involved with delinquent behavior, drugs, and alcohol. Often such youngsters face the prospect of treatment under some duress. This may be mild, such as parental pressure, or severe, such as therapy as an alternative to jail or hospitalization. Doubt is sometimes expressed about the possibility of therapeutic effects occurring under such conditions. Many of the articles in the chapters on antisocial behavior and substance abuse assume that adolescents can benefit from involuntary treatment programs. These efforts require, as an early step, attempts to induce motivation for change. Methods employed to do this range from positive relationship building to increase the therapist's credibility to active confrontation, pointing out the unsuccessful aspects of the antisocial acts. The fact remains that many treatment efforts come to grief at this point.

The preponderance of behaviorally oriented techniques in this book does not imply a downgrading of the importance in our view of the therapeutic relationship in the treatment process. On the contrary, we believe that the quality of the relationship is more crucial to treatment outcome at this stage of life than at any other. An extended consideration of the vicissitudes of the therapeutic relationship is beyond the scope of this book. Two works that address this area are by Donald J. Holmes

(*The Adolescent in Psychotherapy*, Boston: Little, Brown, 1964) and John E. Meeks (*The Fragile Alliance*, Baltimore: Williams and Wilkins, 1974).

Family Issues

Professionals who accept adolescents for treatment must address the issue of the role of the family in relation to the therapist. Regardless of the patient's protestations of independence or alienation from the family, the other family members, especially parents, are affected by changes resulting from the therapy, and they may react in ways that augment or challenge therapeutic gains. It is a frequent clinical observation that changes in a child's condition or symptoms can provoke parents to withdraw the child from treatment at an incomplete or critical juncture. Reasons given may be financial, fear of the child's dependence upon the therapist, and so forth. But an underlying issue may be the parent's role in the child's behavior and their reluctance to examine this role. It is therefore of primary importance that the clinician have a clear sense of how he or she relates in a clinically helpful way to the other family members. A major task for the therapist is to assist the family in supporting and maintaining changed behaviors and relationships.

A range of viewpoints is available regarding how to manage this task, extending from treatment of the family as an indivisible unit to simultaneous separate meetings, with shadings in between. Minuchin, a proponent of the family systems approach, argues that the adolescent should be seen as part of the entire family in treatment (S. Minuchin, *Families and Family Therapy*, Cambridge, Mass.: Harvard University Press, 1974). In his view, when the entire family is in the room, the interrelationships and the family structure, the main elements requiring modification, are easily observable.

M. Sperling (*Psychosomatic Disorders in Childhood*, New York: Jason Aronson, 1978) describes a distinctly different approach. In her work with children and adolescents with severe symptomatology, she conducted simultaneous separate treatment of mother and child—without the child's knowledge of the mother's involvement. She pointed out that the advantages of this method were extensive material necessary for treatment, supplied by the mother; the opportunity to counsel and treat the mother closely; and providing the child with a greatly needed sense of a private, exclusive relationship. Though these two viewpoints are diametrically opposed, both theorists have dealt extensively with the problem of monitoring and therapeutically affecting family issues relating to the teenager's problems.

Steps in Intervention

Effective intervention involves a number of important steps. The first, which we have already alluded to in numerous ways, is the establishment of a therapeutic alliance. Central to the task of establishing this alliance is a task we have not yet discussed—that of defining the problem or problems that will be the focus of treatment. For successful achievement of therapeutic goals, it is necessary that there be some consensus among client, family, and therapist as to what these goals should be and what will constitute evidence that they are being achieved. Haley makes the point that it is the therapist who must accommodate to the family's perception of the problem (J. Haley, *Problem-Solving Therapy: New Strategies for Effective Family Therapy,* San Francisco: Jossey-Bass, 1976). For example, although he or she may see the problem as one of family relationships, the therapist cannot afford to lose sight of the fact that this particular adolescent may be coming for treatment because of failure in school or drinking too much. Amelioration of family relationship problems without a concomitant decrease in these symptoms is not a therapeutic success.

Definition of the problem forms the basis for the development of assessment procedures. Ongoing monitoring of progress is an integral component of behavior therapy approaches, but it is equally important in family therapy and other interventions. It is essential to evaluating whether or not the intervention is succeeding, and it occasionally provides a basis for confronting a client or family with a lack of real commitment to therapeutic change. Mash and Terdal provide comprehensive coverage of techniques of assessment that coordinate well with the problem categories we employ (E. Mash and L. Terdal (Eds.), *Behav-*

ioral Assessment of Childhood Disorders, New York: Guilford Publications, 1981).

The major purpose of this book is to assist the therapist in the next step, that of selecting an appropriate intervention. For each problem covered, we present a variety of intervention strategies. Within the constraints of the relationship with client and family, the therapist must select and implement a strategy of intervention that will have an impact on the referral problems. At the same time, it is necessary to pay attention to weaknesses and vulnerabilities in individual family members and in family interaction patterns that, if left untreated, will lead to the reemergence of problems once the therapy contact has been terminated.

Finally, long-term follow-up is necessary in the treatment of most problems. It is almost never the case that therapy can be terminated with the assurance that all problems have been dealt with effectively and that additional difficulties are unlikely. Follow-up visits are a necessity both from the standpoint of individual patient management and so that the therapist can learn about the long-term consequences of his or her therapeutic interventions.

The procedures reported in this book are effective ways of dealing with specified problems or categories of adolescents in difficulty. Wherever possible, we have collected a variety of procedures for each problem considered; so alternatives can be reviewed and a selection most suited to the people involved can be made. The therapist considering adoption of an unfamiliar technique should first review the full article. Many of these authors refer to important earlier work, which it would also be helpful to review. Our experience is that this supplemental reading offers further understanding of the treatment rationale and considerations of practical application. The choice of procedure, method of offering help, and the decision about when to introduce the intervention—among other aspects—influence and are influenced by the interrelationships among therapist, referred patient, and significant others. For the clinician coming from a background stressing the primacy of the therapeutic relationship, we believe the specialized techniques presented in this book will greatly enhance treatment effects.

1

Emotional Disorders

The American Psychiatric Association's DSM-III treats anxiety disorders and affective disorders as separate categories of disturbance (American Psychiatric Association, *Diagnostic and Statistical Manual of Mental Disorders,* 3rd ed., Washington, D.C.: American Psychiatric Association, 1980). For the purposes of this volume, it is convenient to use the more general heading of emotional disorders and to include under it problems in which anxiety predominates along with those for which depressed mood is the main concern.

Most of the problems included have anxiety as the central feature. This includes fears, anxieties, phobias, obsessions, compulsions, and hysterical reactions. Preventive treatment of minor symptoms as well as treatment of specific disorders typi-

cally involves learning to manage anxiety and tension. A variety
of approaches to treatment is covered, including relaxation
training, cognitive change methods, and implosive therapy. Particularly important is the combined approach advocated by
Meichenbaum, which appears to have applications to more than
one kind of problem.

Depression presents somewhat differently in adolescence
than it does in adulthood (I. B. Weiner, "Psychopathology in
Adolescence," in J. Adelson [Ed.], *Handbook of Adolescent
Psychology,* New York: Wiley, 1980). The young adolescent is
likely to manifest depression through difficulties with concentration, excessive tiredness, and frequent somatic complaints.
Depressive feelings are often warded off by excessive activity.
The older adolescent at times uses drugs or sexual promiscuity
as a means of overcoming depressive feelings. They may not
verbalize the feelings they are experiencing but instead act them
out in uncharacteristic, antisocial, or delinquent behavior. The
treatment approaches recommended for adolescent depression
include encouraging verbal expressions of feeling, modifying depressive thoughts, and setting limits on undesirable behaviors.

Many adolescents suffer with emotional problems that
are not so severe as to warrant a psychiatric diagnosis but are
nevertheless distressing and can significantly affect subsequent
development. Test anxiety, for example, influences level of academic achievement and in an indirect way may ultimately exert
an influence on identity formation. Also, as Weiner points out,
though fewer than 10 percent of all adolescents are diagnosed as
depressed, a large proportion display depressive symptoms in
the form of dysphoric mood, self-depreciation, crying spells,
and even suicidal thoughts. This chapter suggests treatments not
only for specific disorders but also for less severe manifestations
of anxiety and depression, the early treatment of which may
prevent the development of more serious problems.

Fears, Anxieties, and Phobias

Fear is an adaptive response that minimizes exposure to danger. This may be a physical danger, such as that associated with bodily injury, or a psychological one, like that of losing an important person or failing at an important task. Anxieties are more vague than fears. The stimulus is often less clearly defined and the association between stimulus and anxiety response may be symbolic or may even have come about accidentally. When fears are exaggerated or when the connection between stimulus and response involves unconscious symbolism, the reaction is characterized as a phobia. Fears, anxieties, and phobias interfere markedly with normal patterns of living.

Test anxiety is a common problem in adolescence, at times interfering with educational functioning; school phobias may also interfere to a marked degree with academic success; and fears and phobias associated with medical procedures prevent some adolescents from receiving adequate health care. Some anxieties interfere with normal bodily functions like eating and sleeping and others may interfere with normal bodily functions like eating and sleeping and others may interfere with routine daily activities like driving a car or going into a building. Therapies for such problems usually involve weakening the association between a particular stimulus and fearful and anxious responses, though therapy may also involve reducing tensions that are only indirectly related. Reinforcing alternative responses like relaxation and replacing anxiety-generating thoughts with positive self-statements are common approaches to treatment. At times it is also beneficial to explore the unconscious meaning of a particular fear stimulus.

13

Test-Taking Practice Plus Cognitive and Relaxation Training

AUTHORS: S. Little and B. Jackson

PRECIS: Reducing test anxiety through cognitive and relaxation training and improving test performance through practice in test taking

INTRODUCTION: Little and Jackson indicate that the primary problem in test anxiety is worry (negative and unproductive cognitions) that interferes with test performance. Worry includes thoughts like "I can't do this," "I'm going to flunk," "This exam isn't fair," and "We never studied this." The major objective of their approach to treatment is to direct attention away from these irrelevant thoughts and focus it productively on the test-taking task.

TREATMENT METHOD: The treatment described was given to seventh- and eighth-grade students with high scores on a self-report measure of test anxiety. Treatment involved twice weekly group meetings of one hour each for three weeks. On alternate weeks, an audiotaped rationale for treatment that focused on how worry interferes with performance and how it can be controlled by deliberately changing one's thinking was presented. Clients were presented with videotapes of student models successfully overcoming test anxiety and were given practice with academic tasks along with specific instructions to focus attention on the task and inhibit thoughts about self. Reminders to focus attention were gradually replaced with a tone signal prompt, and this was also withdrawn by the last session. Training in muscle relaxation was provided as an aid to focusing attention.

TREATMENT RESULTS: There was a significant reduction in self-reports of both general anxiety and test anxiety. Clients also improved on tests of cognitive functioning. The cognitive improvements appeared to come primarily from practice with test taking rather than from cognitive or relaxation training.

COMMENTARY: This study illustrates that the negative effects on performance of test anxiety can be overcome through simple practice with taking tests and that feelings of anxiety can be reduced through cognitive and relaxation training. The training described involves audio and videotape equipment that may not be available to some therapists; however, it seems likely that most clients could achieve the same effects through verbal instructions and the use of imagery techniques. The addition of training to make positive self-statements might augment the effects that have already been demonstrated.

SOURCE: Little, S., and Jackson, B. "The Treatment of Test Anxiety Through Attentional and Relaxation Training." *Psychotherapy: Theory, Research, and Practice,* 1974, *11,* 175-178.

Cognitive Restructuring Plus Relaxation Training

AUTHOR: D. H. Meichenbaum

PRECIS: Coping with anxiety through relaxation coupled with changes in habits of thinking

INTRODUCTION: Meichenbaum reports that the major causes of poor test performance for test-anxious individuals are failure to attend adequately to the test-taking task and high emotional arousal. He indicates that others have found that test-anxious people spend excessive amounts of time worrying about how they are doing and ruminating about the choices they have to make. He states that they are often preoccupied with feelings of inadequacy, anticipation of unpleasant consequences, and heightened awareness of bodily sensations, all of which interfere with performance. His proposed treatment for test anxiety involves increasing awareness of anxiety-arousing thoughts and

teaching the test anxious person to cope with anxiety by relaxing and by substituting task relevant self-instructions for negative thoughts.

TREATMENT METHOD: Treatment was carried out in groups
over an eight-week period. The initial sessions were devoted to
group discussion focused on each of the following:

   1. The negative self-statements made by group members
during pretreatment testing. (Examples are "I never do well on
tests" or "I bet my friend is already finished with this part.")
   2. Other situations in which the same or similar self-statements are made
   3. The fact that such statements are often irrational and
can trigger feelings and behaviors that lead to poor performance

   In subsequent sessions, clients were taught muscle relaxation and the use of slow, deep breathing to facilitate relaxation,
and the group established a hierarchy of anxiety-arousing events
associated with test taking. They were then asked to visualize
themselves performing the least anxiety-arousing activity in the
hierarchy and coping with whatever anxiety this aroused by
slow, deep breathing and by telling themselves to relax and remain focused on the test-taking task. They were encouraged to
use any self-statements they could think of that would focus
their attention on test taking and inhibit irrelevant thoughts. If
for some reason they were unable to overcome anxiety, they
terminated the image and got back into a state of relaxation before trying again. Once they had anxiety under control, they
moved on to the next item in the hierarchy.

TREATMENT RESULTS: Twenty-one people ranging in age
from seventeen to twenty-five had volunteered for treatment.
Eight of them were assigned to the treatment described. Treatment produced significant improvements in a number of areas.
Grade-point averages improved. Scores on a digit symbol test
improved. Clients reported that not only was anxiety no longer
interfering with performance, but that after treatment, the

anxiety they did experience actually had a facilitating effect on performance.

COMMENTARY: The use of the group modality makes this a highly efficient method for the reduction of test anxiety symptoms. These symptoms not only interfere with daily living, but can also have a lifelong impact in terms of school success and access to career opportunities. The approach used here could probably, with minor modifications, be used to alleviate anxiety in a variety of situations (for example, public speaking or giving a piano recital) where it might otherwise interfere with optimum performance.

SOURCE: Meichenbaum, D. H. "Cognitive Modification of Test Anxious College Students." *Journal of Consulting and Clinical Psychology,* 1972, *39,* 370-380.

A Multimodal Approach to Speech Anxiety

AUTHOR: M. Weissberg

PRECIS: Relaxation, desensitization, and positive thinking in the treatment of speech anxiety

INTRODUCTION: Weissberg, drawing on literature regarding test anxiety, suggests that successful approaches to this problem should also be applicable to speech anxiety. He proposes a treatment based on the work of D. Meichenbaum employing relaxation, desensitization, and anxiety-inhibiting self-statements.

TREATMENT METHOD: Two female college freshmen, enrolled in a speech course, reported intense anxiety and worry whenever they watched speeches being given or gave speeches themselves. Both were treated simultaneously in three two-hour sessions. The initial session was devoted to a presentation of the treatment rationale and to discussion of typical self-statements made by each student in public speaking situations. They reported such statements as "My speech will probably be the worst one in the class," "If I mess up this speech, I'll never pass the course," and "I'm really stupid. . . . Now everyone knows." There was further discussion regarding situations in which similar thoughts occurred. Students were taught to reduce tension through muscle relaxation and through imagining themselves in pleasant, relaxing situations. For homework during the ensuing week, they were instructed to practice relaxation daily and to pay attention to anxiety-arousing self-statements.

In the second session, there was extensive discussion of the illogical and self-defeating nature of these statements. Underlying beliefs regarding such things as the necessity of being liked by everyone were challenged, and the replacement of anxiety-arousing statements with anxiety-inhibiting statements was discussed. The latter included "Even if I blow the speech, that doesn't mean I'm a stupid and worthless person" and "Better take some slow, deep breaths and calm down." In the second half of this session, students were instructed to relax and then to visualize items from a twelve-item hierarchy of anxiety-arousing images. They were taught to eliminate anxiety responses to each image by using positive self-statements and by slow, deep breathing. Beginning with the least anxiety-arousing scene, each was presented for about thirty or forty seconds, followed by a period of relaxation. There were five presentations of each item before moving onto the next. Those items not completed during the second session were worked on during the third.

TREATMENT RESULTS: Self-reported anxiety in speaking, social, and testing situations decreased markedly, and both students rated speech anxiety as "greatly improved."

COMMENTARY: This brief treatment, which has been demonstrated effective for both speech and test anxiety, can proably be used in other performance anxiety situations as well. Larger groups, which are in no way contraindicated, would make it more cost effective.

SOURCE: Weissberg, M. "Anxiety Inhibiting Statements and Relaxation Combined in Two Cases of Speech Anxiety." *Journal of Behavior Therapy and Experimental Psychiatry,* 1975, *6,* 163-164.

Study Skills Training and Desensitization

AUTHORS: R. W. Lent and R. K. Russell

PRECIS: Two multicomponent treatments for test anxiety, each employing study skills training and a variation of desensitization

INTRODUCTION: Treatment of those who suffer from excessive test anxiety involves more than the reduction of anxiety levels. Usually there is a corresponding need to improve test performance. Lent and Russell, in an attempt to meet both goals, devised two multicomponent strategies for the treatment of test anxiety in college undergraduates.

TREATMENT METHOD: Both strategies involved a study skills component with training in how to prepare for a test, along with training in how to take a test. Both also involved learning to control muscle tension through practice in tensing and relaxing various muscle groups. The two treatments differed in their use of relaxation skills to combat test anxiety.

Students in the systematic desensitization and study skills training group were instructed to achieve a state of relaxation and then to visualize items from a hierarchy of anxiety-arousing scenes related to test taking. When the student was able to stay relaxed while visualizing the item lowest in the hierarchy, he or she moved onto the next and so on until all items had been mastered.

Students in the cue controlled desensitization and study

skills training group were taught to pair the cue word "calm" with relaxing so that "calm" became a stimulus for relaxation. Once this connection was established, they were asked to visualize for ten seconds items from a hierarchy of anxiety-arousing scenes associated with test taking and to use the cue word to overcome any anxiety arousal. If they succeeded, they repeated this exercise before moving on to the next item in the hierarchy. If at any time they were not successful, they reestablished physical relaxation before beginning again with that particular item in the hierarchy.

TREATMENT RESULTS: Both treatments were equally effective in decreasing the negative or debilitating aspects of anxiety for college students and in helping them harness anxiety for constructive purposes. Overall anxiety levels were reduced for both generalized anxiety and for anxiety produced in testing situations. Lent and Russell were unable to demonstrate improved test performance on specific tests, but both groups showed improvement in terms of overall grade-point average.

COMMENTARY: Both these treatments can be used effectively to decrease test anxiety and to enhance academic performance. Either could probably be improved by the inclusion of regular practice sessions in test taking. As with most treatments, the feasibility of using the group modality is an important factor in keeping down treatment costs.

SOURCE: Lent, R. W., and Russell, R. K. "Treatment of Test Anxiety by Cue-Controlled Desensitization and Study Skills Training." *Journal of Counseling Psychology,* 1978, *25,* 217-224.

Learning to Use Anxiety

AUTHORS: J. Malec, T. Park, and J. T. Watkins

PRECIS: Modeling and role playing of effective study and test-taking behaviors as a treatment for test anxiety

INTRODUCTION: Not all anxiety is undesirable. Moderate amounts can even facilitate test performance. Malec and his colleagues designed a treatment using both modeling and role playing to teach test-anxious college students to perform effectively while studying and taking tests.

TREATMENT METHOD: Treatment involves only two sessions. During each session, videotaped models who experience test anxiety demonstrate effective coping by focusing attention on task-relevant behavior. Each tape includes three scenes. One shows the model becoming anxious while studying for the test, and the next shows him experiencing anxiety just as the test is about to begin. In each case he refocuses attention on behaviors necessary for success. The final scene reveals that he has succeeded in achieving better than expected performance and shows him receiving positive reinforcement for having handled himself so well. After the videotape presentations, students are split into pairs and given copies of the script to act out. Each student has the opportunity to play both parts in the script.

TREATMENT RESULTS: After experiencing this training, students reported on an anxiety questionnaire that they had learned to use test anxiety constructively, and they commented that this would improve their ability to take tests.

COMMENTARY: This treatment program was quite brief but produced a positive effect. Although all students felt that they had been helped, many reported that the treatment was too short; and it isn't clear whether only attitudes and feelings, as opposed to behaviors and test outcomes, were influenced. Those who use this strategy should probably integrate it with more comprehensive, multicomponent approaches rather than using it as the sole treatment for test-anxious students.

SOURCE: Malec, J., Park, T., and Watkins, J. T. "Modeling with Role Playing as a Treatment for Test Anxiety." *Journal of Consulting and Clinical Psychology,* 1976, *44,* 679.

Brief Treatment of Hemodialysis Phobia

AUTHOR: R. C. Katz

PRECIS: Brief treatment of a hemodialysis phobia using relaxation, desensitization, stimulus control, and social reinforcement

INTRODUCTION: In many cases there is a reality basis for the fear that later becomes an unreasonable phobia. Katz presents a case in which awkward administration of a medical procedure by an inexperienced technician led to a continuing fear and at times even panic wherever the procedure was to be performed in the future.

CASE HISTORY: The patient was an eighteen-year-old male with a chronic kidney problem requiring hemodialysis three times weekly. On the occasion of the patient's first treatment, a student technician failed to insert a vascular catheter properly and had to make a second attempt. The patient became quite fearful that an air bubble would enter his circulatory system and cause serious complications. Fear continued at each successive treatment and at times turned to panic when he was confronted with an unfamiliar or inexperienced technician.

TREATMENT METHOD: Treatment was carried out in a single ninety-minute session. The patient was reassured that his fear reaction was not unusual. It was explained to him that fears are learned reactions and that they can also be unlearned. He was trained in muscle relaxation, and a hierarchy of anxiety-arousing events associated with hemodialysis was constructed. The lowest item in the hierarchy was "waking up on the morning of a scheduled dialysis treatment," and the highest was "having the catheter reinserted." The patient was instructed to visualize each item while completely relaxed, beginning with the lowest item and working gradually toward the highest. Presentations lasted thirty to forty seconds. If anxiety was experienced, the item was repeated after relaxation had been reestablished. No more than two presentations were required for each item. At the end of the treatment session the patient was instructed to continue practicing relaxation at home.

Members of the hemodialysis team were also involved in treatment of the phobia. They were told that for the immediate future treatment should be administered only by experienced technicians with whom no panic attacks had occurred. New staff members were to be introduced gradually by being present for treatments administered by those with whom the patient was familiar. The patient was to receive detailed instructions on the steps involved in hemodialysis and to be prepared for any irregularities that might occur. He was to be praised for undergoing treatment without becoming emotionally upset.

TREATMENT RESULTS: The immediate effect of the ninety-minute treatment session was that the patient could think about dialysis without experiencing emotional distress. In the following months when receiving hemodialysis treatment, he no longer experienced fear or panic or showed signs of being emotionally upset. New technicians were introduced without incident, and even their occasional initial failures at catheterization did not cause undue distress. Over the six-month period of follow-up, there was no recurrence of phobic reaction.

COMMENTARY: The possibility of learned fear reactions to medical interventions is ever present. Anxiety, uncertainty, and pain are natural concomitants of illness and injury. Sensitive staff can usually prevent adverse reactions to treatment through adequate preparation and education of the patient and through relaxed and skillful execution of their duties. When fear reactions do occur, relaxation and desensitization appear to be the treatment of choice for the adolescent patient. The approach outlined by Katz can undoubtedly be applied to adverse reactions associated with a variety of medical interventions.

SOURCE: Katz, R. C. "Single Session Recovery from a Hemodialysis Phobia: A Case Study." *Journal of Behavior Therapy and Experimental Psychiatry,* 1974, *5,* 205-206.

Overcoming Avoidance of Dentistry

AUTHOR: R. K. Klepac

PRECIS: Promoting dental care by reducing dental fears and increasing pain tolerance

INTRODUCTION: Dental fears can be manifest in a variety of ways, including putting off making appointments, emotional reactions during treatment, and complete avoidance of dental visits. All those young people about whom Klepac reports were avoiding treatment, and none had seen a dentist within the preceding three years.

CASE HISTORY: All five clients were in their late teens or early twenties. None was able to comply with even the simple request that they seek a dental check-up (no treatment to be provided) prior to enrolling in the behavioral treatment program. The goal of treatment, agreed to by all clients, was that they be able to get through a series of dental appointments and return to the dentist for a six-month follow-up visit.

TREATMENT METHOD: In the first session the rationale for

treatment was given and all procedures to be used were explained. A dental fear survey, which included ratings on the degree to which various dental treatment stimuli evoked discomfort and indications of the client's usual response to those stimuli, was administered. There were also open-ended questions
regarding previous dental experiences. On the basis of information obtained during the first session, a hierarchy of fears was
constructed. Appointments were scheduled three times each
week, with initial treatment sessions devoted to relaxation
training. It took from eight to twelve sessions for each client
to reach the point where he or she could quickly and easily relax at will. At this point the hierarchy that had been constructed in the first session was reviewed, and modifications
were made as needed. Practice in visualizing neutral scenes was
provided, and following this, another series of twice weekly sessions was devoted to eliminating the anxiety associated with
each item in the anxiety hierarchy. The client was instructed to
relax and then to imagine the item lowest in the hierarchy.
When he or she was able to maintain relaxation while visualizing
this stimulus, the next item was introduced, and so on until all
were mastered. This took from twelve to twenty sessions. During the final session, instructions were given to continue daily
practicing of relaxation and to use this skill to eliminate any
tension resulting from subsequent dental treatment. Dental appointments were made and follow-up on whether they were
kept was ensured by requiring a $50 deposit that would be re-
turned only when follow-up assessments were completed.

In attempting to follow through with dental treatment,
two clients decided that low pain tolerance was the main problem and that their fears were entirely warranted. Treatment to
increase pain tolerance involved presentation of a series of
shocks to the nonpreferred forearm. The initial intensity was
0.5 mA, and the series proceeded in increments of 0.5 mA to
the point where shock was "definitely painful." The client
then relaxed before receiving a second series, which began three
steps below the maximum for the last series and proceeded until
the client requested it to be terminated. This procedure was repeated two more times, each time beginning three steps below

the previously attained ceiling. Following each series, the client was praised for progress. Six sessions, each consisting of four shock series, were enough to make it possible for both clients to achieve the original goal of completing dental treatment and returning for a six-month checkup.

TREATMENT RESULTS: Three out of five clients succeeded in overcoming their fears sufficiently to complete dental treatment and to return for a six-month dental checkup. The other two required the additional course of pain tolerance treatment.

COMMENTARY: Clearly defined goals and flexibility in adding a new treatment component made it possible for all clients to achieve success. As many as thirty sessions were required to reach this point; but, considering the fact that clients had to overcome fears concerning a situation in which pain was actually being experienced, this does not seem excessive. The method utilized to guarantee follow-up data made it possible to obtain data on all clients. Without such a method the additional treatment needs of two clients might never have been discovered.

SOURCE: Klepac, R. K. "Successful Treatment of Avoidance of Dentistry by Densensitization or by Increasing Pain Tolerance." *Journal of Behavior Therapy and Experimental Psychiatry*, 1975, *6*, 307-310.

Management of Phobias Through Implosive Therapy

AUTHOR: A. F. Fazio

PRECIS: Decreasing fears associated with medical injections through the use of implosive therapy

INTRODUCTION: Implosive therapy involves presenting the

client with anxiety-arousing stimuli at maximum intensity while preventing escape and avoidance behaviors. The goal is for the client to learn that the fear stimulus is in fact harmless or at least considerably less harmful than previously imagined. A secondary goal is to diminish the power of all associated stimuli to evoke anxiety, thereby increasing the client's freedom of thought and behavior.

CASE HISTORY: The client was a twenty-year-old female who presented with a phobia regarding medical injections. She reported that her phobia was "spreading" in a way that greatly restricted her freedom. In theaters and auditoriums, she experienced anxiety if she could not sit at the end of the row, positioned to escape if anything frightening came on the screen. She claimed she would leave school or quit her job rather than submit to a health examination.

TREATMENT METHOD: Treatment was initially focused on halting the spread of anxiety. The client was asked to imagine a professor in a classroom who pierced his ears in a brutal and gory manner in front of the class. She was told to imagine that her friends forced her to look at him and prevented her escape. She was then told to imagine him piercing her ears. The more upset she became, the more vividly the anxiety-arousing material was described. Toward the end of the session, such images had lost their power to upset her.

In subsequent sessions, scenes involving injections were presented, and free associations yielded related anxiety stimuli as well as psychodynamic symbolism underlying specific fears. As hypotheses were developed regarding feared unconscious impulses (for example, violent impulses toward siblings), the acting out of these impulses was also presented in vivid imagery. As various scenes lost their power to elicit anxiety, the client was encouraged to go out of her way to expand the number of associations to anxiety stimuli and to focus attention of anxiety stimuli encountered outside the treatment situation.

TREATMENT RESULTS: After twenty-one sessions, the client reported having allowed her physician to prepare her for a blood test without actually injecting her, and after twenty-three sessions, she was able to tolerate receiving a blood test without fainting. MMPI scores that had previously been abnormal were at second testing all within the normal range. At twelve-month follow-up, the client reported observing and receiving blood tests without becoming anxious.

COMMENTARY: Although implosive therapy can be effective, it is certainly riskier than other forms of treatment for anxiety. It requires an experienced clinician to make judgments about a particular client's emotional resiliency and ability to tolerate anxiety. The therapist must have a thorough knowledge of psychodynamic theory and be well qualified to deal with uncontrolled anxiety reactions.

SOURCE: Fazio, A. F. "Implosive Therapy in the Treatment of a Phobic Disorder." *Psychotherapy: Theory, Research and Practice*, 1970, 7, 228-232.

Relaxation and Desensitization in Treatment of Nightmares

AUTHORS: A. J. Cellucci and P. S. Lawrence

PRECIS: Behavior therapy to reduce frequency and intensity of nightmares

INTRODUCTION: Many people experience nightmares, although they are usually not a chief reason for therapy referral. It is not clear if nightmare sufferers have more psychological problems than others or whether their sleep pattern seriously affects their daily behavior and adjustment. The use of several procedures, sometimes including medication, has reportedly been helpful in alleviating nightmares. In this article, a systematic desensitization procedure was employed.

TREATMENT METHOD: College undergraduates who reported having nightmares twice a week or more were recruited. They were asked to record occurrence and subjective intensity of each nightmare. Major anxiety-provoking dream material was also noted, to be used in constructing "anxiety hierarchies." The first training session involved explaining desensitization in theory and application. Relaxation training was also begun. The anxiety-provoking dream images were ranked by each person in order of increasing upsetting effect.

The standard desensitization procedure calls for the client to achieve relaxation and to remain relaxed while visualizing first mildly provoking, then increasingly disturbing scenes. Clients were assisted in constructing and rank-ordering such scenes based on anxiety-arousing dream images, and they were taught two ways in which anxiety might be reduced. They could repeat part or all of the relaxation procedures, or they could change the image, imagining a scene in which they coped very well with the threatening situation. Another option was to repeat to themselves that this was just a dream. They were advised to try to relax when imagining each new scene, but not to persist for more than a minute. If they could not relax, they were to return to the previous item in the hierarchy. The goal was for clients to learn that relaxation is incompatible with anxiety and can reduce the frequency and severity of anxiety-provoking thoughts.

TREATMENT RESULTS: Those in the treatment group showed a greater decline in number and intensity of nightmares than did members of a control group. In those people who were contacted for one-month and seven-month follow-ups, these gains were, on the average, maintained or increased, with few or no nightmares being reported.

COMMENTARY: This study was conducted with undergraduates, presumably including late adolescents, however this procedure seems worth considering for adolescents of all ages. There is didactic material as well as a structured training program. Nightmares are frequently reported by therapy patients, and unless these patients clearly show secondary benefit from having or reporting nightmares, they may be willing to attempt this straightforward procedure.

SOURCE: Cellucci, A. J., and Lawrence, P. S. "The Efficacy of Systematic Desensitization in Reducing Nightmares." *Journal of Behavior Therapy and Experimental Psychiatry*, 1978, *9*, 109-114.

Family Contracting for Sleep Disturbance

AUTHORS: E. M. Framer and S. H. Sanders

PRECIS: Indirect treatment of disturbed sleep by behavioral improvement of family communication

INTRODUCTION: This report describes the reduction of sleep disturbance by resolution of family problems. Behavioral contracting was applied to overcome communication deficits. An unusual feature of this successful intervention was that no causal relationship between referral problem and family communication difficulty was identified. Furthermore, the referral problem improved without direct treatment.

CASE HISTORY: Len's mother was quite concerned with his episodes of sleep disturbance. They seemed to come about four times a week and might consist of sleepwalking, sleeptalking, verbal outbursts, thrashing about as if in combat, and so forth. There had been a recent upsurge in frequency of these behaviors, apparently associated with increased friction between Len and his parents. Len himself was minimally concerned about his sleep habits, having little recall in the morning. He was, however, motivated to improve relations with his parents and to improve his skills in negotiating with them for privileges.

Five weeks of baseline recording by his mother showed that from zero to three episodes of sleep disturbance occurred each week. The model developed by Patterson and his associates (G. R. Patterson, *Families,* Champaign, Ill.: Research Press, 1971) was used in treatment. Sleep problems were not addressed. Instead, privileges desired by the boy were discussed and behaviors necessary to earn privileges were negotiated. Therapist assistance resulted in "if-then" contracts at each session. After six sessions, the family continued to practice contracting by themselves. A follow-up session was held after a five-week interval.

During the contracting-with-help phase, Len's sleep problems rose sharply at first, then declined to none by the end of these meetings. By final follow-up, one year later, almost no further indications of sleep disturbance were seen. Len and his parents reported better communication and an improved relationship generally.

COMMENTARY: In this successfully treated case, no causal relation between the treated behavior and the referral problem was discussed. The rationale for selecting communication problems for treatment was that these might be important stressors for the boy; however, he had not been previously motivated to receive help for this. No difficulties were described in getting the parents to collaborate on this alternative problem. It is probably advisable to look for such concurrent stressors in all youngsters referred for other specific complaints.

SOURCE: Framer, E. M., and Sanders, S. H. "The Effects of Family Contingency Contracting on Sleeping Behaviors in a Male Adolescent." *Journal of Behavior Therapy and Experimental Psychiatry,* 1980, *11,* 235-237.

Additional Readings

Cavior, N., and Deutsch, A. "Systematic Desensitization to Reduce Dream-Induced Anxiety." *Journal of Nervous and Mental Disease,* 1975, *161* (6), 433-435.

Having a recurring dream of violence made this sixteen-year-old male quite anxious. He had it at least weekly. Scenes were related to violence he had actually observed at home. A modified systematic desensitization program reduced the troubling anxiety, but not the frequency of the dream. Relaxation was taught and a twelve-step anxious scenes hierarchy was constructed. The major change in the desensitization procedure was that the patient did not repeat the entire relaxation sequence after completion of each step in the anxiety hierarchy. Instead, the therapist simply suggested the patient was still relaxed. The patient was upset during the first session, but by the third expressed confidence that anxiety would no longer be a problem. Anxiety was still minimal at six-month follow-up.

Hall, R. A., and Dietz, A. J. "Systematic Organismic Desensitization." *Psychotherapy: Theory, Research and Practice,* 1975, *12,* 388-390.

Hall and Dietz report on the simultaneous treatment of three phobias (fear of heights, fear of driving, and fear of being in classrooms) through the desensitization treatment of a single phobia involving fear of choking. Careful analysis of hierarchies associated with the three phobias suggested that all were related to a disturbance in inner ear functioning. The patient was indeed found to have a chronic inner ear infection that might at times stimulate a gag reflex. Desensitization of a hierarchy of items related to fear of choking led to long-term relief of the three phobias with which this client initially presented.

Hampe, E., Noble, H., Miller, L. C., and Barrett, C. L. "Phobic Children One and Two Years Post Treatment." *Journal of Abnormal Psychology,* 1973, *82,* 446-453.

These authors report on long-term follow-up of brief intensive treatment for phobic children. The two treatments studied were reciprocal inhibition therapy and psychodynamic therapy.

The following conclusions emerged: (1) The type of treatment appeared to be less important than the fact of receiving some kind of psychological treatment. (2) Younger children showed more dramatic improvements than older children. Phobias generally go away within about two years, even if not treated, but treatment hastens recovery.

Haynes, S. N., and Mooney, D. K. "Nightmares: Etiological, Theoretical and Behavioral Treatment Considerations." *The Psychological Record,* 1975, *25,* 225-236.

    The three studies reported include a trial of implosive therapy with college students, among them late adolescents. Four women had histories of one to five nightmares weekly for several years. Nightmare themes included physical or sexual assault, rejection, or fears of these (none of this had ever happened to them). Six weekly one-hour implosive therapy sessions were held. The client reported the previous week's nightmares for the first twenty minutes. She then listened to the therapist's effort to depict an emotionally charged scene using the themes she had reported. Scenarios of rape, robbery, assault, and emotional rejection were described at length. Most women reported being anxious, breathed heavily, and looked tense during the descriptions, though one took four sessions to feel or show any response. All reported reduced number and severity of nightmares, with gains tending to remain at three-month follow-up.

Kaplan, R. M., McCordick, S. M., and Twitchell, M. "Is It the Cognitive or the Behavioral Component Which Makes Cognitive-Behavior Modification Effective in Test Anxiety?" *Journal of Counseling Psychology,* 1979, *26,* 371-377.

    The contention of Kaplan and his colleagues is that Meichenbaum's cognitive-behavioral treatment for test anxiety is effective only because of its cognitive component and not as a result of desensitization (see Meichenbaum, "Cognitive Restructuring Plus Relaxation Training," in the present section). To test this hypothesis, they randomly assigned students to various conditions, including one that replicated Meichenbaum's treatment and one that included only the cognitive manipulations. Results suggest that with a strong cognitive component, desensitization may not add anything to the overall treatment effect. Unfortunately, different outcome measures were used in the two studies; so results are not directly comparable.

Le Unes, A. L., and Siemsglusz, S. "Paraprofessional Treatment of School Phobia in a Young Adolescent Girl." *Adolescence,* 1977, *12,* 115-121.

The authors report on the treatment of a fourteen-year-old school phobic girl through intensive involvement with a paraprofessional volunteer. In the beginning, the volunteer drove the girl to school each morning, taking a roundabout tour designed to help her to become more relaxed. When fears lessened, the morning ride was replaced by an after-school meeting to review the events of the day. In addition to working to decrease anxiety, the volunteer also engaged in a variety of activities designed to build self-confidence. Her efforts were supported in a limited way through group and individual therapy. Treatment resulted in dramatic improvement in school attendance and academic functioning.

Vaal, J. J. "Applying Contingency Contracting to a School Phobic: A Case Study." *Journal of Behavior Therapy and Experimental Psychiatry,* 1973, *4,* 371-373.

Vaal describes the case of a thirteen-year-old boy who had resisted school attendance for six months. The first step in treatment involved intensive interviews with parents and school personnel. No good explanation for school avoidance could be found. A list of behaviors desired by parents and school personnel was developed, including such items as "coming to school on time without tantrum behavior," "attending all classes on schedule," and "remaining in school until dismissal time." It was worked out with the boy that various privileges that he had been enjoying would become contingent on his meeting his responsibilities. Parents were kept informed on a daily basis concerning class attendance. After having missed most of his classes for the first six months of school, the boy attended without absence for remaining six months and returned to school without incident in the fall semester.

Obsessions and Compulsions

An obsession is a repetitive thought; a compulsion is an internal pressure to carry out some behavior repeatedly. Obsessive thoughts can consume increasingly large proportions of one's thinking, leading to loss of performance in other spheres of activity. Although a single event may be the original source of the thought, its reccurrence may be set off by an increasing number of stimulus situations. Compulsions are often maintained by fears of dire events if the behavior is not performed. Like obsessions, they may become more complex and pervasive. Learning theory treatments may be cognitive as well as behavioral. An example of a cognitive approach is to help the adolescent find a justifiable need for the compulsive act and then to create a better way of meeting that need. The strategies presented here attempt to minimize the strength of the irrational stimulus or to maximize the client's ability to control associated problem behaviors.

Behavioral Treatment of Obsessional Thought in a Young Adolescent

AUTHOR: L. M. Campbell III

PRECIS: Disruptive thoughts eliminated by a modified thought-stopping technique

INTRODUCTION: Thought-stopping techniques have proven effective with adults in interrupting and reducing persistent, undesired thoughts or fantasies. Modification of the usual procedure was undertaken in the case of this early adolescent.

CASE HISTORY: John ruminated increasingly on his sister's awful death, which he had witnessed nine months previously. Bloody and disfigured, she had died in his arms. His thoughts of her and the incident soon severely affected him in many areas, including eating, sleeping, and schoolwork.

Baseline data on daily number and duration of episodes were obtained. By the time he was referred for help, ruminative periods had increased to over a dozen per day, each lasting about twenty minutes. The therapist tried to discover what started each obsessive period, only to find that, at that point, unrelated events were setting them off.

TREATMENT METHOD: The therapist elicited from John a number of pleasant thoughts or fantasies. John was trained to evoke the upsetting ruminations at will and to stop them by loudly counting backwards from ten to zero. At zero he was to start thinking about a pleasant fantasy. When this procedure was mastered, the next step was to repeat it, subvocalizing the counting. After this, John was ready to carry it out in public without disrupting others. He was told to practice every night and to keep a record of the number and extent of ruminative events. His mother was to keep notes on his behavior as well.

TREATMENT RESULTS: By the second session, daily ruminations were down to three, and by the fourth session, John reported no episodes for the prior week. Treatment was considered successful, and there were no more visits. Follow-up three years later revealed no resumption of negative thoughts. Other behavioral problems had ceased, and John was a serious student with an active social life.

COMMENTARY: Thought-stopping techniques have gained wide acceptance, being simple and effective. The quasi-ritual element of "countdown" introduced by Campbell is a minor but useful addition that might appeal to a younger person. For the older adolescent, thought stopping can be useful, although the ritualistic methods may not be necessary.

SOURCE: Campbell, L. M. III. "A Variation of Thought-Stopping in a Twelve-Year-Old Boy: A Case Report." *Journal of Behavior Therapy and Experimental Psychiatry*, 1973, *4*, 69-70.

===

Behavioral Treatment of Rituals

AUTHOR: D. Green

PRECIS: A three-part treatment program with relaxation, habituation, and cognitive procedures

INTRODUCTION: Adolescence is a time when many poorly functioning obsessional styles are first noticed by others. Early treatment seeking is a favorable prognostic sign. Behavior therapy stressing response prevention is useful with compulsive behavior. This procedure alone is less useful with upsetting cognitions and related mood disturbance. Behavior, feelings, and thoughts were all targets for change in the program used here.

CASE HISTORY: Fifteen-year-old Paul experienced peremptory urges to check or repeat acts. He would think that if he failed to do so, harm, perhaps death, would come to family members. These thoughts, plus great physical tension and flushed face, would be quickly relieved when he completed a ritual. Drug therapy (chlorimipramine) had been only temporarily effective. Paul was able to identify four additional special problem areas: stereotyped touching of objects, repetitive passing through doors at home, stereotyped placing of a tea cup, and leaving his school desk. Examination of family dynamics yielded no useful information.

TREATMENT METHOD: A three-stage treatment approach was used. The first stage was *autogenic training*. This is a structured relaxation training program developed by J. H. Schultz. Notable features of this procedure include autosuggestive instructions. Paul learned to follow the format closely to relax deeply in five sessions.

The second stage was *satiation*. The goal here was habituation, becoming accustomed to the emotional upset caused by the obsessional thought. Repeated presentation of the upsetting thought made that thought less threatening. First the therapist helped Paul to put the thought into precise language. Paul then relaxed deeply and attempted to focus on the obsessional thought, repeating it to himself. He indicated when he could hold the thought and practiced until he could do so calmly for five minutes. Three sessions were needed for this phase. That satiation was attained was proved when Paul reported the disturbing thoughts were becoming hard to hold, seeming to "fade."

The third stage was *response prevention*. The rationale for this step was that when urges are externally prevented, the force of the urge often abates. Although family and friends are natural assistants in blocking reported urges in daily life, Paul decided to do all response prevention himself. He exerted himself to stop all checking behavior. Two sessions were devoted to planning and implementing this phase.

TREATMENT RESULTS: Paul used this program well. The

structured autogenic relaxation, known to be attractive to compulsives, appealed to him. He quickly learned that relaxing was an effective blocking agent for disturbed thoughts. During the satiation phase, he discovered that thinking was much easier because anxious disruptions were fewer. His checking behavior had decreased notably before response prevention was introduced and remained at minimal levels. His mood improved, and all target behaviors were notably diminished. At six-month follow-up, his gains had been maintained. His obsessional style was largely unchanged, but was no longer a problem. He held the relaxation training in high regard, continuing daily use.

COMMENTARY: This multistage model was well suited to the presenting problems. Autogenic relaxation and satiation were notably effective. Usefulness of response prevention was less clear because the rituals were already reduced before this phase began. We agree with Green's point that this procedure appeals to the obsessive-compulsive patient and to the patient with especially strong need to control the treatment.

SOURCE: Green, D. "A Behavioral Approach to the Treatment of Obsessional Rituals: An Adolescent Case Study." *Journal of Adolescence*, 1980, *3*, 297-308.

Self-Imposed Behavior Restriction of a Compulsion

AUTHORS: A. D. Poole and G. C. Bodeker

PRECIS: Gradual reduction of compulsive behavior by a stepwise, externally set time limit

INTRODUCTION: For patients who understand that their compulsive behaviors reduce anxiety, there is little relief in this knowledge. They feel the burden of tension if they try to refrain from the undesired habit. Usual procedures aim at anxiety reduction, but there are alternatives. *Time restriction,* used in a structured manner, is sometimes sufficient to reduce the extent of compulsion.

CASE HISTORY: A late adolescent girl reported that she had to rock in a chair before bedtime or else she could not sleep. She looked anxious and bit her nails during the initial interview. She was doing well socially and academically. Her only request was for help in stopping the rocking. She was instructed to note the time spent rocking each night and seen two weeks later. At that time, the information indicated a mean of twenty-five minutes of rocking, with a range of ten to fifty-six minutes. She received reassurance that she could learn to gradually control this.

TREATMENT METHOD: An agreement was reached that for the next two weeks she could rock at will up to 25 minutes (the baseline mean). Over this period, data she reported showed an average of 9.6 minutes, with a range of 0-25 minutes. Encouraged, she then accepted a maximum of 20 minutes per night for the next three weeks. She continued to reduce mean rocking time and reported more nights of no rocking. By the time the maximum of 10 minutes was set, she had stopped.

TREATMENT RESULTS: Over the following two months she rocked once, when she was physically ill. When followed up six months later, she reported no recurrence of rocking. She had in the meantime adopted a habit of taking a few minutes to straighten her room and prepare for next day's school. The time spent on this appeared to be appropriate.

COMMENTARY: This technique is not a direct anxiety reduction procedure. Why it works is a matter of conjecture. The authors wonder if rocking increased anxiety for this student, so that the task was actually reduction of anxiety-provoking behavior. Our view is that because this youngster was able to exercise self-control in other places, the task was teaching her to extend self-management to this problem area. Learning to control a behavior previously thought unmanageable is in itself a powerful anxiety-reducing event. This procedure may be appropriate with adolescents who are involved in authority struggles with parents and therapists.

SOURCE: Poole, A. D., and Bodeker, G. C. "Using Time Restriction to Modify Compulsive Rocking Behavior." *Journal of Behavior Therapy and Experimental Psychiatry*, 1975, *6*, 153-154.

Additional Readings

Friedmann, C. T. H., and Silvers, F. M. "A Multimodality Approach to Inpatient Treatment of Obsessive-Compulsive Disorder." *American Journal of Psychotherapy*, 1977, *31*, 456-465.

A severely incapacitated eighteen-year-old was hospitalized with complaints of counting and walking rituals when family therapy proved unhelpful. He was also greatly depressed. His history showed an isolated life-style. Behavior techniques, family, and milieu therapy were used as well as individual psychotherapy. A three-phase model was employed: assessment, behavior targeting and modification, and discharge planning. The patient kept a diary of obsessional thoughts, a paradoxical technique. Thought stopping was successfully employed. At discharge, more anxiety was reported, but obsessive-compulsive behavior was reduced. With therapy, his anxiety and obsessive-compulsive behavior was minimal at two-and-a-half year follow-up.

Lindley, P., Marks, I., Philpott, R., and Snowden, J. "Treatment of Obsessive-Compulsive Neurosis with History of Childhood Autism." *British Journal of Psychiatry*, 1977, *130*, 529-597.

A seventeen-year-old male was hospitalized for extreme

obsessive-compulsive behavior. His history included a diagnosis of childhood autism. He had rituals, could not make decisions, repeatedly checked himself, and was compulsively slow. A token economy system was employed, giving rewards for achieving target goals. Specific techniques included response prevention, exposure in vivo, modeling, and a social skill program that utilized role rehearsal, reversal of roles, and videotaped feedback. He also received medication. Postdischarge brought improvement and then relapse. Failure of family and postdischarge residences to continue the operant program were seen as the major problem. Long-term community support was felt to be necessary.

Mastellone, M. "Aversion Therapy: A New Use for the Old Rubber Band." *Journal of Behavior Therapy and Experimental Psychiatry,* 1974, *5,* 311-312.

The client with a ritual is instructed to wear a large rubber band on the wrist. After committing the problem habitual act or when feeling the urge to do so, the band should be snapped. This is not necessarily painful, but can interrupt undesirable behavior sequences. It also serves as a cue for control or alternate behaviors. Hair pulling, homosexual fantasies, overeating, and intrusive thoughts are some behaviors the author has treated with this aid, with varied results. For treatment programs requiring a cueing procedure, this maneuver might be useful.

Weiner, I. B. "Behavior Therapy in Obsessive-Compulsive Neurosis: Treatment of an Adolescent Boy." *Psychotherapy: Theory, Research and Practice,* 1967, *4,* 27-29.

A fifteen-year old boy developed several rituals, together with feelings that terrible things would happen to his family or himself if the rituals were not performed. Weiner focused on the ritualistic behaviors, with the goal of reducing their intrusive effect. He assisted the boy in naming a positive rational reason for a ritual. The goal was accepted by the therapist, and the next step was to agree on simpler, less time-consuming methods to achieve the goal. The boy used the substitute rituals, and reported lessening of ritual behavior and anxiety, with fewer overwhelming urges. On followup he reported he had given up both the regular and the substitute rituals.

Hysterical Reactions

Adolescents with hysterical reactions display extremes of emotional sensitivity and a wide range of associated behavior problems, including respiratory, muscle, or sensory difficulties for which no organic basis is found. Identifying the hysterical component is made more difficult by the fact that emotional instability is a predictable part of adolescent development. An unusual feature that may be present is a relative lack of concern with the symptom or its effects. In addition to psychoanalytic psychotherapy, behavioral treatments of these symptoms may be employed, including relaxation (sometimes aided by hypnosis), reinforcement of behavior incompatible with the symptom, and introduction of expectancy of change. The studies included in this section report behavior that may indicate a hysterical process but focus exclusively on the presenting conversion symptom.

Treatment of an Hysterically Contracted Muscle

AUTHORS: E. M. Hendrix, L. M. Thompson, and B. W. Rau

PRECIS: Elimination of muscle clenching by relaxation and changed environmental reinforcement

INTRODUCTION: The behavioral treatment of hysterical symptoms focuses on what currently reinforces and thereby maintains the problem behavior. From a variety of severely disturbed behaviors, the target selected was the one about which the family expressed most concern. An interesting feature of this case is the parents' concentration upon a single symptom, ignoring other serious problems.

CASE HISTORY: After a minor bruise, a fourteen-year-old girl complained of increasing numbness in her arm. Following this, her right hand clenched into a fist following a similar injury and remained chronically tight. She was not doing well in school, compared to her more gifted siblings. Generally seen as "sickly," she made numerous complaints that led to many school absences. Hospitalized for evaluation, she was transferred to a psychiatric ward after her arm was pronounced medically clear. Assessment showed she got several positive responses to her "injury": staying home from school for several weeks, decreased fighting by parents, and lessened criticism of her mother by her father. However, the symptom bothered her parents sufficiently for them to agree to the hospital evaluation. The parents resisted all inquiries into family dynamics; so a direct treatment program was developed.

TREATMENT METHOD: The girl's fingers were wrapped around a dynamometer, and it was demonstrated that she grew gradually fatigued. She was taught relaxation and told that this would help her to relax her hand and keep it relaxed. To control parental support of the symptom, a contract was arranged as follows: The girl would remain in the aversive environment (hospital) until her hand was open twenty-four hours. Then she could transfer to a day hospital, with full discharge after seven days with an unclenched hand. To earn any more than one weekly parental visit, her hand would have to remain open one minute.

TREATMENT RESULTS: The symptom was greatly relieved in the first session, with her hand open after twenty minutes of relaxation and suggestions to remain relaxed. She moved quickly to the final goal of discharge. No relapse occurred during the treatment phase, and no clenching had occurred by the time of a follow-up telephone call nine months later.

COMMENTARY: This case provides a clear procedure for the relief of hysterical symptoms involving tensed muscles. The description of the patient shows that only one behavior that fit this diagnostic category was treated; several others she showed could not be addressed due to parental resistance. The authors acknowledge the need for more extensive effort to broaden parents' understanding of the problem. At the earliest possible point, explanations and recommendations need to be made. It is clear from follow-up information that the "hysterical" syndrome was not affected. New somatic problems emerged to receive similar parental reinforcement. With such extensive effort, including hospitalization, directed at the one symptom, reluctance to acknowledge the seriousness of the child's problem may prove an insuperable obstacle.

SOURCE: Hendrix, E. M., Thompson, L. M., and Rau, B. W. "Behavioral Treatment of an 'Hysterically' Clenched Fist." *Journal of Behavior Therapy and Experimental Psychiatry,* 1978, *9*, 273-276.

Treatment of Writer's Cramp

AUTHORS: M. Arora and R. S. Murthy

PRECIS: Relaxation and extensive retraining exercises

INTRODUCTION: This case combined two procedures effectively to treat a muscle difficulty that had no physical origin.
Some features of the conversion pattern were present, although
further information would have been helpful to confirm a diagnosis. The behavioral procedure employed had several advantages. It was obviously related to the specific complaint, easily
learned, and did not require the use of avoidance procedures.

CASE HISTORY: After eighteen months of increasing difficulty, a nineteen-year-old male requested help with his inability
to write. No precipitating events were recalled. Hand movements
had become rigid, making writing slow, more difficult, and fa-
tiguing. As the problem became worse, the young man took to
holding his pen in his fist and was able to write a little this way.
He did not report anxiety before or during writing or look upset
while writing. The problem was worse in the presence of others,
however, and he was concerned about its effect on his ability to
hold a job. He had already turned down one job because of the
writing requirements.

TREATMENT METHOD: The patient was first taught a relaxation procedure. Second, he was given exercises to be performed
with the hand in a supinated position (arm out, palm facing up-
ward). When relaxation had been learned, a watercolor paint
brush was given him, and he was shown how to grip it with fingers straight and thumb holding it in a relaxed grip. In daily
one-hour sessions, he relaxed for the first half hour and then did
exercises with his hand in the position previously described.
First he drew large (10 cm) circles slowly, taking care to remain
relaxed. As he reported comfort with this, he was asked to draw
smaller circles, and then spirals and lines. The next step was to
hold the brush as he would hold a pen and draw large capital

letters. He then repeated the sequence, beginning with large circles, with a soft pencil. After he began to write two and three little words, a sketch pen and then an ordinary pen were employed until he could write continuously without tension for up to a half-hour.

TREATMENT RESULTS: At six-month follow-up, the patient was doing well at a job requiring ten to twelve pages of handwriting daily.

COMMENTARY: The authors' use of relaxation is consistent with other work in relief of similar symptoms. There are several alternate explanations for the improvement that was obtained. Among them are the authors' notions of the effects of relaxation and retraining as well as the possibility that loss of reinforcement for the problem behavior during the long procedure led to its decline. Also, the length of the program may have introduced a mildly aversive element into the situation. Writer's cramp, though rare, is a serious problem; so the availability of a successful technique is welcome.

SOURCE: Arora, M., and Murthy, R. S. "Treatment of Writer's Cramp by Progression from Paint Brush in Supinated Hand." *Journal of Behavior Therapy and Experimental Psychiatry,* 1976, 7, 345-347.

Additional Readings

Armstrong, H., and Patterson, P. "Seizures in Canadian Indian Children: Individual, Family and Community Approaches." *Canadian Psychiatric Association Journal,* 1975, *20,* 247-255.
   Hysterical seizures were related to strongly conflicting cultural pressures in an epidemic of seizures among thirteen observed children between eleven and eighteen. In small, remote

Indian settlements of this type, normally indulged children and adolescents were attracted to a high consumption life-style by media presentations, only to realize that their inadequate skills and education made this status unreachable. The "fits" followed a clearly described pattern, gaining great attention for the individual. Episodes occurred at times of excessive drinking by the father or intolerable fighting by parents and resulted in the parents' cessation of this upsetting behavior. Parental counseling helped to ease tensions. Reduction of reinforcing factors such as attention and physical contact was encouraged. More social activities by the community were encouraged to give better outlets for attention seeking. The result was a major reduction in hysterical seizures.

Gross, M. "Pseudoepilepsy: A Study in Adolescent Hysteria." *American Journal of Psychiatry*, 1979, *136*, 210-213.

In a two-year period this clinic saw nineteen adolescents with psychogenic seizures, fourteen girls and five boys. Thirteen of the nineteen had first received a diagnosis of epilepsy and had been referred only after failure to respond to treatment. Sixteen received a diagnosis of hysterical neurosis (two were called schizophrenic and one, borderline). Underlying conflicts were identified in fifteen (89 percent). Once organic causes were ruled out, insight or supportive therapy, sometimes with neuroleptic or antidepressant medication, was the most preferred treatment. Hypnotherapy was also frequently employed.

Munford, P. R., and Chan, S. Q. "Family Therapy for the Treatment of a Conversion Reaction: A Case Study." *Psychotherapy: Theory, Research and Practice*, 1980, *17*, 214-219.

In this study, a conversion reaction of incessant eructation was treated as an operant, subject to learning theory approaches. Behavior oriented family therapy was used to treat a fourteen-year-old girl whose burping had increased sharply within the past sixteen months. She had a long history of physical illness and irrational fears. Evaluation showed problems of separation, independence, and handling of sexuality. The family was told the symptom was without medical origin and reflected a family problem. The girl was asked to record her burps at chosen daily intervals. Agreements were made for her to do chores and receive praise for them. Less burping meant more opportunities for activities outside the home. Other contracts were made within the family and between the husband and wife. Within four weeks, the burping had decreased and did not return within two years. The contingency contracting resulted in a broad range of improved family interactions.

Rathus, S. A. "Motoric, Autonomic and Cognitive Reciprocal Inhibition in a Case of Hysterical Bronchial Asthma." *Adolescence,* 1973, *8,* 29-32.

A twenty-two-year-old woman had begun having breathing difficulty after her mother's death from cancer. Attacks followed stress periods. At the start it was proposed to her that she was imitating her mother's gasping for air as a response to stress. Because this was learned, training in competitive responding was done. Next she received relaxation training and was told to commence this every time an attack began. She was instructed to try to welcome each attack as another chance to prove she could control it. She gave the attacks a pleasant masculine name to help her greet them. The fear of not getting enough air during an attack disappeared immediately. Her relaxation became increasingly automatic. Her awareness of attacks decreased. At termination (after six sessions), she was advised to expect spontaneous recurrence and to welcome them. Only two incidents occurred under stress in two years, and these were successfully controlled.

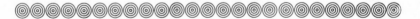

Depression

Depression is perhaps the most frequently reported complaint heard by therapists. It may be a separate problem of serious proportions or just one of many factors in another problem syndrome. Sometimes it is a normal, time-limited response to disappointment and losses. It may also be, suggests Sugar, a part of the adolescent developmental process, resulting from the giving up of childlike security in the drive for separation and independence.

Emotionally, sad or blunted feelings are reported. There may be a component of anger, sometimes shown in accusations of inadequate treatment or uncaring loved ones. Expressions of lowered self-worth or reduced ability or expectations from others are common. Energy level is also lessened. Suicidal potential is markedly greater (for therapy strategies with seriously suicidal adolescents, see Chapter Seven). The therapy approaches here range from psychoanalytic to behavioral. Treatment may be broadly directed or narrowly focused on troublesome symptoms. Improved self-directed activity, a more realistic acceptance of one's situation, and more satisfactory relations with people are frequently cited features of successful treatment.

Focusing on Depressive Consequences
of Normal Adolescent Maturation

AUTHOR: M. Sugar

PRECIS: Understanding the stages of psychic loss and adaptation efforts

INTRODUCTION: An early task in treatment is to distinguish between serious pathology and the more usual, stormy, stage-appropriate adolescent problems. Sugar argues that some depressive behavior in teenagers should be viewed as a sign of developmentally appropriate mourning. Adolescents pass through three stages of mourning the loss of infantile, internalized fantasy representations ("objects") of parents. Giving up the closeness and dependence implied in these objects is a necessary step to adulthood.

The earliest of the stages in depressive mourning is labeled the *separation-protest* phase. The beginning of attempts to separate onself from parental objects is marked by fears and clinging, with alternate episodes of hostility and fleeing. Loss of the object leads to anger-related attempts to restore the unrecoverable former state. Absence of a parent complicates this phase; separation from an absent person is more upsetting. The therapist can help parents to understand their child's tentative movements toward psychological apartness as a sign of growth.

By the time of the teenager's progression to the *disorganization* phase, some minimal acceptance of the loss of the old relationship exists. Aimless and restless behavior, anxiety, and complaints of not understanding parents or one's own behavior are noted. One hears expressions of hope for better adjustments, and there are attempts to find alternatives to reunion with the lost object. Sugar views antisocial behavior occurring at this time as a sign of extended object mourning. For parents, the problem is that adolescents may react badly both to their overprotective support or restoration of earlier relationships as well as to a rapid release of external control.

The *reorganization* phase, arriving in late adolescence, is less turbulent. Relational problems, one sign of attempting to cover for the object loss, are explored with peers of both sexes. There is concern with fulfilling one's potential. There may be frequent retreats to the prior disorganization phase, and the reorganization phase can extend into the mid-twenties.

TREATMENT METHOD: For some teenagers, treatment of depressive elements is similar to assisting them to pass through a mourning of their loss of childhood dependency. Therapists help to bring out expressions of loss and depression-related feelings, which can release the patient to return to better functioning. The range of interventions, including counseling parents, brief or extended therapy, and hospitalization, follows an assessment of the severity of the behavioral difficulties shown. This in turn relates to the stage of the adolescent's mourning, extent to which help is needed to pass through this phase, and any uncommon traumatic life events.

COMMENTARY: This article illustrates the viewpoint that many emotional and behavioral difficulties of adolescents stem from efforts to accomplish developmental tasks of this period. The problems may be normal; yet the youngster may need help that peers cannot provide and that will not be accepted from parents. Assessment of type and extent of depression may be clarified by considering the developmental tasks being attempted by the teenager.

SOURCE: Sugar, M. "Normal Adolescent Mourning." *American Journal of Psychotherapy*, 1968, *22*, 258-269.

Therapy of Depression Related to Absence of Parental Authority

AUTHOR: H. J. Friedman

PRECIS: Reestablishment of standards and goals necessary for adolescent development

INTRODUCTION: Friedman describes the consequences of abdication of authority by parents in matters of limits and values. This article is included in this section because of the prominence of depression in the three case examples presented. It should be remembered, however, that many problems occur when parents fail to set standards or respond to their children's noncompliance.

The authority or parental surrogate role is sometimes employed by the therapist if the adolescent is behaving in a self-endangering manner. Friedman suggests wider use of this role where parents abandon their limit-setting responsibilities or side with their adolescent children's rebellion on social-ills grounds. Therapist limit setting may help, assisting in a corrective experience. The therapist takes a stand, firmly keeping to a view stressing growth goals and performance standards.

CASE HISTORY: Referred by a psychiatrist, Richard, sixteen years old, described his depressive and hopeless feelings as too much to bear. He was a high school senior and blamed his problems entirely on school difficulties, saying that an excessive work load made him nervous. His parents, he said, were concerned that overwork might cause a breakdown. He asked what the doctor thought of his plan to leave school.

The doctor knew Richard had been drinking heavily and on a daily basis, once to the point of unconsciousness. Both parents had psychiatric histories, related, they believed, to overwork. Richard appeared better adjusted than his four siblings. The doctor noted that Richard received more restrictions and was sought for chores, but his parents avoided his more hostile brothers.

TREATMENT METHOD: The doctor would not accept Richard's wish to be declared unfit for school or the service. His intelligence and work abilities were pointed out, and the pressing need to apply to colleges was noted. Richard was surprised and resisted this. The comment was made that applying for a college and being accepted was not binding. Further, the therapist suggested that good decisions were not always made when people were depressed. The moment of decision was a year away, and a year's perspective might lead to a different outlook. The boy's low estimate of his chances was interpreted as reflecting his feelings of worthlessness. His attempts to justify his problems and reluctance to work were similarly challenged. Complaining of assigned readings, he responded to a suggestion by reading on his own with surprised pleasure. He negotiated with teachers, finding them surprisingly flexible.

TREATMENT RESULTS: He was accepted at a strict college, elected to go, and continued treatment on a monthly basis. His academic performance was excellent, and he reported mastery of continuing impulses to drop out.

CASE HISTORY: Ann, sixteen years old, traced her depression to social problems at school, where she was noticed for her promiscuity and drug use but couldn't talk to her peers. Her divorced father still considered himself boss at her home and viewed her behavior as morally repugnant. Her mother liked counterculture living and was permissive.

TREATMENT METHOD: The therapist helped Ann to view her behavior from a nonmoralistic basis. Ann used the therapist's stand that her depression was related to feelings about her behavior to establish some control over her acting out.

    Failure to learn was also a source of depression. Her mother and the school taught that learning happened only when it was fun. Her father took the opposite view. The therapist, again taking a middle view, acknowledged the rewards of effort. The therapist's push to consider college was also counter to the philosophy of taking time to "find" herself. He took a stand against her plans to drop out.

TREATMENT RESULTS: Ann later attended a college, received all As, and looked around for a more challenging school.

COMMENTARY: This approach is warranted, in Friedman's view, for these adolescents who seek treatment and who are able to acknowledge a need for values in their lives. Such an approach helps adolescents who have been allowed excessively to express the passivity and regression that is a common adolescent defensive retreat. These adolescents accepted nonauthoritarian confrontation and disagreement. The therapist's willingness to take a stand rather than avoid conflict was a key element in success. Family therapy sessions directed toward clarifying roles and improving communication would probably also be beneficial in such cases, particularly for families with younger adolescents.

SOURCE: Friedman, H. J. "New Considerations in the Treatment of Certain Adolescent Patients." *Adolescence,* 1974, *9* (34), 155-168.

Cognitive Therapy for Persisting Depressive Feelings

AUTHOR: W. G. Johnson

PRECIS: Coverant control therapy for depressive thoughts not influenced by behavior change

INTRODUCTION: In spite of major behavior improvement, sometimes depressive feelings persist. Johnson bases his treatment for continuing depression on the coverant model of Lloyd Homme. Coverants or cognitive statements influence and can be influenced by managing their relationship to behaviors. The effect of coverants upon target behaviors is altered by carefully arranging their relations to one another. For example, following the Premack principle, a low-probability, desired thought can be made to occur more frequently by pairing it with performance of a frequently occurring act. Two cases described in this article show how coverants affect behavior and vice versa.

CASE HISTORY: Don, seventeen years old, had made progress in four therapy sessions. Presenting problems had included limited social skills and fear of staying on the college campus on weekends. He had begun to date and was able to make some small talk and to remain on campus on weekends. Depressive episodes, however, interrupted these positive steps. Morning blues would result in avoidance of the rest of the day's schedule. He would call his parents and usually received a sympathetic hearing. Instructions were given that instead of calling his parents, he should carry out one of the new activities that had become enjoyable to him. This had only a brief positive effect.

TREATMENT METHOD: The coverant intervention was intended to increase occurrences of positive self-statements by requiring that they precede instances of a high probability behavior, that of urination. Don was required to carry a set of index cards in his pocket, each one with a description of positive change he had made. Until they occurred without prompting, Don read a card to himself each time he was about to urinate.

TREATMENT RESULTS: He did this six to ten times a day and did not need the cards after several days. His depressive episodes ceased after two weeks of this regimen, and he started to experience spontaneous positive thoughts.

COMMENTARY: This case illustrated the use of behavior to change coverants whose strong effects had remained a problem. Also reported here was a procedure (used with an adult but apparently applicable to adolescents) that changed behavior by use of coverants. Writings from diverse viewpoints caution clinicians to assess both behavior and nonbehavior aspects (such as thinking, mood, and self-esteem) in evaluating the extent to which depression has lifted. In this article, a follow-up report would have been helpful. The theoretical rationale for the procedure is well grounded and the method can be appealing to the client. For problems of negative cognitions, this method should be considered.

SOURCE: Johnson, W. G. "Some Applications of Homme's Coverant Control Therapy: Two Case Reports." *Behavior Therapy*, 1971, *2*, 240-248.

Therapy of Adoption-Related or Alienated Depression

AUTHOR: K. M. Tooley

PRECIS: The antidepressant effects of establishing better links to past and future

INTRODUCTION: The author describes what she believes is an emotional survival skill: ability to hope. She suggests this is based on a sufficiently effective connection to one's past self. When an adolescent's past self-recreation is fostered by fond parental recollections, it provides support for his or her hope of a similarly enjoyable life in the future. Suicidal depression may reflect a lack of hope that things could be different.

Tooley talks about the "inner treasury" of hope-sustaining elements amassed in childhood. These include special possessions (items evoking fond memories), shared memories, and stories of early childhood. These elements support a positive sense of having been cherished in the past. The adolescent may be partly protected against alienation by hope of reviving this sense of being cherished and bringing pleasure to people again some time in the future.

With adoptive parents, the question "where did I come from," understandably anxiety provoking, is often answered in an excessively factual way. Tooley argues that this query contains a second, hidden question, "where am I going?" The implication is that the adolescent is concerned with fantasies of both past and future living possibilities. Additional problems also arise when the child is adopted. Parents may be anxious about revealing sensitive information in a damaging manner.

They are advised to give bits of information that the child can weave into daydreams. For example, national origin and any achievements of natural parents may be shared, if thoughtfully censored. An edited story would describe a natural father as mechanically skillful, but conceal the fact that he had been a safecracker. While on the subject of characteristics, it is wise to comment on the child's own talents and promise, supporting future-directed thinking and fantasizing.

An additional resource for a growing young adolescent is others' recollection of early events in life that he or she does not personally remember. This again supports attempts to construct images of future success as a loved person. For those patients whose parents cannot recall their early years, clarifying the loss in therapy brings little relief.

Therapists may help adolescents develop strengths to cope with depressive feelings. Part of the therapist's task is to reinforce the available positive connections to personal and family "inner resources." Strengthened associations to these positive earlier experiences can evoke appropriate narcissistic resources that can increase one's investment in the future.

COMMENTARY: The chronically depressed or alienated youngster's therapist can use individual therapy, intensive counseling of parents, or both to aid the child's recovery or construction of a loved self. Tooley's assessment is that the adolescent may make good use of the recovered signs of affectionate consideration by others, even during the drive to become separate from the family. Parents counseled in this manner may feel relieved and supported. (For more discussion of assistance to adoption-related emotional problems, see Pannor and Nerlove, Chapter Three).

SOURCE: Tooley, K. M. "The Remembrance of Things Past:
On the Collection and Recollection of Ingredients Useful in
the Treatment of Disorders Resulting from Unhappiness,
Rootlessness and the Fear of Things to Come." *American
Journal of Orthopsychiatry*, 1978, *48*, 174-182.

Additional Readings

Anthony, E. J. "Two Contrasting Types of Adolescent Depression and Their Treatment." *Journal of the American Psychoanalytic Association*, 1970, *18*, 841-859.

    Anthony's depression categories are a depression with pri-
marily preoedipal features and a more oedipally based syndrome. The preoedipally based adolescent depression, marked
by a symbiotic maternal relationship, shows marked orality and
dependency, narcissistic object relationships, and weak self-
esteem. The patient described was extremely demanding and
evoked considerable countertransference feeling. The second
type has a harsh superego, shows more guilt, and may describe
feelings of loss and emptiness. For this second type, aggressive
thoughts toward ideal parents are redirected inward. The case
example for this type features a markedly parental transference.

Berlin, I. N. "Some Implications of the Development Processes
for Treatment of Depression in Adolescence." In A. P.
French and I. N. Berlin (Eds.), *Depression in Children and
Adolescents*. New York: Human Sciences Press, 1979.

    Berlin reminds us that in Eriksonian terms, the issues of
adolescence are identity versus role diffusion and intimacy versus isolation. Stated as developmental tasks, the goals are
achievement of greater psychological independence, an increasing sense of self apart from the nuclear family, involvement
with a work or career effort, and more successful attachments
with the opposite sex. Progress and regression in these direc-
tions are the rule, and absence of visible stress is not always a

good sign. A case example describes a fifteen-year-old girl with a controlling and manipulating style, hospitalized after a suicide attempt. After progressing well, she sharply regressed. Whereas much prompting had been given before, this time she was not pushed. The staff felt that her new status was such that they did not have to struggle with her to show that her progress was worthwhile. Within a week she returned to her new gains. Berlin suggests that progress followed by regression makes possible a new look at old patterns, without the need for the old interpersonal conflicts.

Catanese, R. A., Rosenthal, T. L., and Kelley, J. E. "Strange Bedfellows: Reward, Punishment and Impersonal Distraction Strategies in Treating Dysphoria." *Cognitive Therapy and Research*, 1979, *3*, 299-305.

Each of several strategies successfully reduced depression over a month-long period. Gains were generally maintained when followed up twenty-four to thirty months later. The treatment involved two thirty-minute sessions, during which the rationale was explained and homework assignments were given. Treatment alternatives were to do one of the following when feeling blue: visualize pleasant scenes; do some brief, pleasant task; mentally scold oneself; perform a mildly aversive but necessary chore; or, at random times, thinking about a broad issue not closely related to one's problems. The authors speculate that two factors common to all methods may have been the major contributors to the general success: distraction from one's preoccupation and learning to assert oneself to do something, perhaps something different.

Kaufman, B. "Object Removal and Adolescent Depression." In A. P. French and I. N. Berlin (Eds.), *Depression in Children and Adolescents*. New York: Human Sciences Press, 1979.

Kaufman offers suggestions on depression related to the striving for autonomy that leads to the deidealization of important figures (notably parents) during adolescence. Kaufman calls this "object removal." It evokes early experiences of loss in people who are used to relating to others primarily as a means of having needs gratified. As the adolescent patient deidealizes his or her parents and acts with increasing independence, the therapist may have to assist in the development of positive but changed relationships between patient and parents. Kaufman describes the case of a fourteen-year-old depressed boy with a history of physical illness. Therapeutic goals, within a dynamic psychotherapy framework, were to help him understand the reasons for his dependency and to help him accept his ambivalence about independence strivings.

Lee, J. A., and Park, D. N. "A Group Approach to the Depressed Adolescent Girl in Foster Care." *American Journal of Orthopsychiatry,* 1978, *48* (3), 516-527.

Depression is common in foster children, stemming from identity and identification dilemmas related to familial losses. Foster children feel anger at the parents who gave them up and at their unvalued self. Girls considered to need a place to work with these issues were referred by caseworkers to a voluntary group. The girls reported that they hated the designation of foster child. They challenged how much workers really cared and what they could do to help because they couldn't return them to their mothers. Help for their anger and grief came from shared discussion. The worker accepted expressions of rage and helped to clarify issues related to acknowledging help from foster parents and workers. Relief from depression was evident with the emergence of more problem-solving activity. The year-long group helped the girls to relate more warmly to others and to be more productive in school.

2

Physical Disorders

Among the psychological problems that present during childhood and adolescence, there is a large group of what can best be categorized as "physical disorders." These include disturbances in eating, eliminating, sleep, and motor movements. For all these disorders there are psychological factors that influence onset, frequency, and severity of symptoms. Eating disorders, for example, have their roots in the early mother/child relationship, and they are often influenced by ongoing family interactions. Faulty toilet training may predispose a child to enuresis, and psychological trauma often triggers onset. Insomnia is tied to worry and tension, and tics are functionally related both to stress and to positive consequences in the form of attention.

A combination of family and behavioral therapies is the approach most likely to be effective for all these problems. Clear definition of target behaviors and systematic manipulation of consequences are important elements in treatment. Families must be involved in eliminating precipitating stimuli as well as inadvertent reinforcement of unwanted behaviors. Direct counseling is often not sufficient, and behavioral change does not take place without careful restructuring of family interaction patterns. In many cases, verbal psychotherapy that clarifies motivations and motivational conflicts is a necessary prerequisite to more specific interventions. Likewise, for those adolescents whose physical problems are related to avoidance of normal peer group activities, social skills training may be a necessary adjunct to treatment of presenting problems. Each of the problems discussed in this chapter requires an individualized approach, and often a mix of several strategies is necessary to bring problem behaviors under control and to promote a healthy adolescent adjustment.

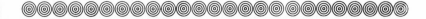

Obesity

Obesity may be defined as higher-than-expected body weight for age, height, and sex; or it can be defined in terms of the amount of fat stored in a particular part of the body, for example, in the triceps folds. The causes of obesity remain uncertain. There is some evidence for an inherited predisposition to being overweight, but there is also evidence to suggest that parents train their children to overeat by overfeeding in the early childhood years. Individual differences in activity level that are present from earliest infancy are also importantly related to the development of excess weight. Although there is confusion about causes, there is little argument about effects. Obese individuals are at increased risk for a variety of physical health problems, including cardiovascular diseases, and they are also much more likely than their normal weight peers to suffer from a variety of psychological problems, including low self-esteem and social isolation. Treating obesity involves changing eating and exercise habits in such a way that there is a proper balance between energy intake and expenditure. Nevertheless, a direct approach is not always the most productive; and it is sometimes necessary to begin treating such problems as low self-esteem, lack of social skills, and fears about growing up before progress can be made in changing eating habits. The therapist who can help the obese teenager overcome the complex of problems with which he or she is likely to present makes an important contribution to adolescent development.

Self-Concept and Weight Management

AUTHORS: S. Stoner and M. Fiorillo

PRECIS: A group treatment approach leads to improved self-concept and weight reduction for overweight adolescent girls

INTRODUCTION: Overweight teenagers often feel depressed, have a negative opinion of themselves, and feel helpless about overcoming their problems. Stoner believes that therapy programs for these adolescents should strongly emphasize improving the way they feel about themselves.

TREATMENT METHOD: Therapy participants were all overweight high school girls, ranging in age from fifteen to eighteen. Treatment involved weekly sessions of one hour each with a therapist selected at least in part for her ability to provide a positive role model. The major emphasis in therapy meetings was on personal grooming and social skills. There were seven major topics: skin care and cosmetics, hair care and styling, clothing selection and alteration, speech and voice control, posture, exercise, and social graces. Each session also included time for discussion of such important issues as sex, dating, and problems with parents. The weight loss component was low key. Girls were given information about specific foods to avoid and about how to plan low calorie menus, and they were encouraged to change their eating habits accordingly. They were weighed each week and their progress was charted.

TREATMENT RESULTS: In sixteen weeks of therapy they all lost weight, and most group members developed a greater sense of personal worth and a more positive view of themselves physically. Weight loss ranged from four to nineteen pounds. One-month follow-up revealed no weight gain and some additional weight loss ranging from zero to seven pounds.

COMMENTARY: It appears that weight loss programs for teenage girls need not focus directly on weight loss and in fact may be more effective when they do not. Although regular monitoring and feedback provide structure, helping the girls look better and feel better about themselves may provide the motivation, confidence, and sense of hope they need to tackle the difficult problem of changing their behavior. Certainly the fact that this approach reduces the likelihood of power struggles about eating behavior increases the likelihood that it will be successful. The program might be further enhanced by a component focused on training clients in the use of positive self-statements.

SOURCE: Stoner, S., and Fiorillo, M. "A Program for Self Concept Improvement and Weight Reduction for Overweight Adolescent Females." *Psychology*, 1976, *13*, 30-35.

Group Behavior Modification

AUTHORS: G. Zakus, M. L. Chin, M. Keown, F. Hebert, and M. Held

PRECIS: Educational and behavior modification approaches combined within a group therapy context

INTRODUCTION: After reviewing the literature on obesity, Zakus and her colleagues concluded that inadequate knowledge about diet and poor eating habits were major problems for the obese adolescent. They decided that by combining educational and behavior modification approaches within a group therapy context they would have the best chance of overcoming these obstacles to weight loss. They also provided a group educational experience for "significant others" whose support would be particularly important to their adolescent clients in changing their eating habts.

TREATMENT METHOD: Treatment was carried out in a health

care setting as one of the activities of the adolescent clinic. Ten girls volunteered, but only five followed through with treatment. These girls were anywhere from 74 to 136 pounds overweight. They met for an hour and a half on Saturday mornings for twenty-five consecutive weeks. Daily records of food intake and the circumstances of eating were maintained, and these were discussed at each weekly meeting. Weights were recorded and graphed. Girls were taught to control specific events that precipitated eating. General rules that were applied to all group members included not buying problem foods, confining eating to one place, not eating while engaged in other activities, slowing down the eating process, and actively controlling distressing thoughts that served as a stimulus for eating.

Each girl's diet was designed by a nutritionist and stressed adequate intake of meat and dairy products, increased intake of low caloric fruits and vegetables, and decreased intake of starches, fats, and sweets. Girls had to be taught to eat a nutritionally sound breakfast, a meal all of them routinely skipped.

TREATMENT RESULTS: It took several months for regular attendance and group cohesiveness to develop. Three of the girls lost weight (from 5.5 to 11 pounds), and the average loss for the total group was 2 pounds. This compared favorably with an average gain of 13.4 pounds over the six months preceding treatment and an average gain of 8.1 pounds for the four dropouts from the program who continued to attend the adolescent clinic.

COMMENTARY: Some weight gain is to be expected during the adolescent period; so even holding the line is an accomplishment, and slow but steady losses are desirable. The approach outlined here does achieve that effect for some girls, but can be improved upon. More systematic reinforcement of desirable behaviors would be the single most important improvement. Rewards for eating appropriate breakfasts or confining eating to one place could be attained with relative ease, and success in attaining them would help clients who often feel at the mercy of their impulses to gain a feeling of being in control. This could be strengthened even further by regular rehearsal of positive statements about self-control.

SOURCE: Zakus, G., Chin, M. L., Keown, M., Hebert, F., and Held, M. "A Group Behavior Modification Approach to Adolescent Obesity." *Adolescence*, 1979, *14*, 481-490.

Comprehensive Treatment for the Obese Adolescent

AUTHORS: J. B. Saffer and G. L. Kelly

PRECIS: Treating the psychological concomitants of adolescent obesity as part of a total weight management program

INTRODUCTION: Saffer and Kelly, although concerned about the physical health aspects of obesity, are even more concerned about its psychological concomitants: low self-esteem, social isolation, excessive dependency on parents, and failure to master the normal tasks of adolescent development. They see the likelihood of a particularly painful and perhaps failed adolescence for obese youngsters unless the problems of obesity are dealt with in a comprehensive fashion.

CASE HISTORY: Fifteen boys and girls ranging in age from thirteen to fifteen participated in the program. All had been evaluated medically before being accepted. The therapy group met as part of each weekly clinic session, and about seven of the fifteen youngsters were generally present. Initially, all showed a striking lack of social and verbal skills. A cohesiveness and concern about each other slowly developed. The focus in therapy sessions went from a "getting to know you" phase to one in which there was considerable group preoccupation with physical complaints and fantasies about accidents and death. Only

gradually was a strong inhibition about expressing anger overcome. Verbalizations of anger gave way to good-natured mutual
teasing and then to constructive problem solving. Discussion of
heterosexual interests emerged quite late in this sequence.

TREATMENT METHOD: Treatment consists of three major
components: diet consultation, an individualized exercise program, and group therapy. Diet consultation involves brief meetings twice monthly with the dietician. The focus is on demonstrating the relationship between food intake and weight gain
and on promoting a sense of personal responsibility about food
intake. The recreational therapist plans an exercise regimen that
he supervises on a weekly basis and maintains weight records,
including photographs taken every four months. The focus in
group therapy is on sharing thoughts and feelings about common problems, overcoming passivity and becoming more competitive, and improving social skills with members of both sexes.

TREATMENT RESULTS: All seven teenagers who participated
regularly lost some weight and one lost thirty-six pounds. The
authors concluded that the acquisition of verbal and social skills
that occurred was even more important than the weight loss.

COMMENTARY: The psychological concomitants of obesity
in adolescence are well known. Saffer and Kelly have described
an approach to dealing constructively with these problems. A
comprehensive approach to adolescent obesity involving this
kind of assistance along with a more behaviorally oriented approach to exercise and eating behaviors would probably be an
even more effective intervention. Other approaches to social
skills deficits that might also be helpful are detailed in Chapter
Three this volume.

SOURCE: Saffer, J. B., and Kelly, G. L. "Treating the Obese
Adolescent." *The Psychiatric Forum*, Fall 1974, *4*, 27-32.

A Developmental Perspective
for Overeating

AUTHOR: C. I. Steele

PRECIS: Important diagnostic considerations in the management of obesity in adolescent girls

INTRODUCTION: Steele provides a developmental rationale for problems of overeating in adolescent girls. She emphasizes the fact that the adolescent task of relinquishing parents as a primary source of emotional support is often difficult and points out that disengagement from parents frequently leads to at least temporary depression. Overeating can be seen as an attempt to overcome such feelings and make oneself feel better. In most cases depression and overeating are transitory symptoms that resolve spontaneously or with brief psychotherapy; however, for some, overeating is only the most obvious sign of a pervasive inability to master the tasks of normal adolescent development. Steele strongly urges that the therapist consider these issues before embarking on a course of therapy.

Steele indicates that when overeating is only the "typical" adolescent reaction to disengagement from parents, it is usually of short duration and does not lead to excessive weight gain. When treatment is required, the client generally takes the initiative in attempting to lose weight and does not come for treatment simply as a result of adult coercion. Those whose overeating is a sign of a more serious developmental problem show a consistent pattern of overeating in response to stress, a lack of initiative in losing weight, and little evidence of movement toward age-appropriate activities and relationships. Diagnostic interviews or testing are likely to reveal signs of serious mental disturbance.

CASE HISTORY: Terry was a fifteen-year-old girl who came for therapy at the insistence of her mother. She was five feet four inches tall and weighed 176 pounds. In addition to her problems with obesity, she showed a pattern of deteriorating school performance and withdrawal from peer group activities. In therapy Terry showed little inclination to discuss her eating problems; instead, she tended to focus on generalized fears about growing up. She showed an obvious desire to remain "her parent's little girl."

Carol was also fifteen years of age. She was five feet two inches tall and weighed 160 pounds. Her parents made the appointment for therapy because of Carol's concerns about being overweight. She was a successful student and had many girlfriends. She had not begun dating but was concerned about being physically attractive. In therapy, Carol initiated discussions regarding eating patterns and also talked freely about concerns that she might have trouble coping with adult roles and responsibilities. In the group Carol found reassurance that others were having similar thoughts and feelings.

TREATMENT METHOD: For girls like Carol, Steele recommends brief individual therapy followed by a group therapy experience. The focus is generally on such issues as lack of self-confidence and uncertainty about growing up. Group therapy provides an opportunity to discover that others have similar concerns. Participants feel confidence in problem solutions backed by group consensus. For the more disturbed adolescent like Terry, Steele recommends individual or family therapy. She does not go into specifics regarding therapeutic strategies, but does indicate that focusing primarily on weight loss is likely to be counter-productive.

TREATMENT RESULTS: Therapy with Terry was unsuccessful, and Steele attributes this to the fact that the therapist failed to make her fears about growing up the central focus of therapy and instead exerted subtle pressures for weight loss and age-appropriate behavior.

Despite the fact that weight loss was not a central focus in group discussions, Carol left therapy having lost thirty pounds.

COMMENTARY: Disengaging from parental attachments and assimilating sexual impulses are important tasks at adolescence. Steele alludes to such concerns in the case material she presents.

Difficulties in either area can cause tension, and the child who has been trained to respond to tension with eating will have difficulty with weight control during the adolescent period. For some adolescents the demands of this period may bring to light more pervasive disturbances. Failure to master the tasks of previous developmental periods has left them poorly equipped to cope with the complexities of adolescent development, and weight loss is not their central concern. For them, therapy should be directed toward developing specific coping skills in areas where they are experiencing stress. Family interviews will probably bring to light ways in which other family members interfere with normal development and reinforce maladaptive behaviors.

SOURCE: Steele, C. I. "Obese Adolescent Girls: Some Diagnostic and Treatment Considerations." *Adolescence,* 1974, *9,* 81-96.

Additional Readings

Chisholm, D. D. "Obesity in Adolescence." *Journal of Adolescence,* 1978, *1,* 177-194.

Chisholm summarizes research on psychological causes and consequences of obesity and describes approaches to counseling and psychotherapy. The orientation is primarily psychodynamic. Chisholm indicates that adolescents most in need of psychotherapy are those with faulty body image, low self-esteem, passivity, overdependence on parents, withdrawal from activities, and social isolation. He also recommends psychotherapy for adolescents whose obesity is reactive to psychological stress.

Cohen, E. A., Gelfand, D. M., Dodd, D. K., Jensen, J., and Turner, C. "Self-Control Practices Associated with Weight Loss Maintenance in Children and Adolescents." *Behavior Therapy,* 1980, *11,* 26-37.

Cohen and her colleagues report on research concerning

the maintenance of weight loss achieved through participation in a pediatric weight loss group. An important correlate of weight loss maintenance was the amount of exercise in which the client engaged. Also important was the extent to which the client took responsibility for self-regulation through self-monitoring of food intake, self-praise for weight control, self-restriction in tempting situations, and self-initiative in increasing activity levels to counteract weight gains. In families of weight gainers, parents took responsibility for these functions but in fact were unable to control either eating or exercise activities adequately.

Magrab, P. R., and Papadopoulou, P. L. "The Effect of a Token Economy on Dietary Compliance for Children on Hemodialysis." *Journal of Applied Behavior Analysis,* 1977, *10,* 573-578.

Problems with diet management can be particularly critical for teenagers with chronic illness. For those with kidney problems, diet compliance can be assessed indirectly by monitoring weight gains and blood levels of nitrogen and potassium. Assessments can be made each time the patient comes for hemodialysis. Providing rewards for achievement of acceptable levels with respect to these variables led to improved weight control and to better control over nitrogen and potassium levels for those who previously had problems in these areas.

Stults, H. "Obesity in Adolescents: Prognosis, Etiology and Management." *Journal of Pediatric Psychology,* 1977, *2,* 122-126.

Stults provides an excellent summary of recent literature on prognosis, etiology, and management. He indicates that behavior modification can be effective in the control of overeating and underexercising. He stresses the need for providing stimuli and resources for personal growth in other areas of living and cautions against an exclusive focus on the control of overeating.

Anorexia Nervosa

Anorexia nervosa is a condition involving excessive self-restriction of food intake that generally has its onset in adolescence. It is characterized by weight loss of at least 25 percent of normal body weight and refusal to maintain a minimum normal weight for age and height. The causes are unclear, but there are often associated fears about becoming fat and distortions in self-perception regarding size and weight. The vast majority of individuals with this disorder are females, and they are frequently amenorrheic. Treatment is complicated because patients typically do not see themselves as having any problem requiring treatment and because struggles for autonomy and control are often a part of the underlying psychodynamics. Treatment planning must take into account failures to master developmental tasks from periods prior to adolescence as well as current difficulties with respect to eating habits, self-perception, specific fears, and family dynamics. Treatment generally involves both crisis management and long-term therapy and follow-up.

Inpatient Therapy

AUTHORS: N. Rollins and A. Blackwell

PRECIS: In-hospital management of severe anorexia nervosa through combined, individual, and parent group therapy

INTRODUCTION: Anorexia nervosa is a condition in which disturbances in eating lead to serious weight loss. Eating disturbance is generally manifest in excessive dieting, but sometimes there is excessive eating followed by vomiting. Dieting is usually precipitated by a fear of being fat. Other symptoms include withdrawal from peer relationships and immature or regressive behavior in relation to parents. Anorexia nervosa frequently has its onset in the transition period between childhood and adolescence, and it has been suggested that it is a defensive reaction by an individuals unable to cope with the stresses and demands of adolescence. Family dynamics in such cases often include power struggles between parents and child and parental blocking of steps toward increased maturity. Rollins and Blackwell divide treatment into two major phases. The first is directed toward reestablishing normal eating patterns and managing family interaction problems, and the second is directed toward promoting insight into the unconscious motivations that have led to the anorexic crisis. Only the first phase is discussed in this article.

CASE HISTORY: Gerry was ten and a half when she first manifested symptoms of anorexia nervosa. She had had a somewhat difficult course of development up until that point. She had a history of breathing difficulty dating all the way back to infancy. During her early school years this problem, coupled with frequent colds, resulted in many days of absense. She had difficulty with schoolwork and with peer relationships and was jealous of her younger sister, who was successful in both these areas. She obtained the attention and affection of which she felt deprived through illness.

Gerry was initially treated on an outpatient basis, but ultimately was unable to cope with the demands of a normal school day. Once admitted to the hospital, she attempted to take charge, engaging in arguments about how long she would have to stay and the frequency of parental visits; and she manipulated parents and hospital staff into conflict with each other. The central concept of this method of inpatient treatment is labeled "holding." This covers a variety of manipulations designed to guarantee the constancy of the child's emotional environment. It involves such actions as setting firm limits regarding eating behaviors and family contacts and accepting resulting anger in a calm manner. It involves managing contacts between parent and child in such a way that each is protected from the others' anger and manipulation until they can learn how to communicate appropriately. It involves coordinating interdisciplinary communication so that the child gets a consistent message from all staff and so that staff have a forum for working through the frustrations and anger that such patients inevitably provoke.

Holding in this case required working out a compromise among staff after Gerry convinced pediatric house staff that she should be sent home. It also involved supporting parents in setting limits and in recognizing and constructively using the anger that they felt at being manipulated. After Gerry was helped to recognize that her breathing problems often occurred in situations where she felt angry, she went on to talk about fears and resentments she had harbored since early childhood. After two and a half months of inpatient therapy, her eating behavior had improved enough so that Gerry could go home. The next phase of treatment involved family counseling and outpatient psychotherapy for Gerry.

TREATMENT METHOD: The method described is for those cases in which serious threat to life, extreme regression, or severe disturbances in the parent-child relationship make outpatient treatment dangerous or impractical. Separate therapists are used for parents and child, with the child's therapist coordinating interdisciplinary communication. A major focus in the therapy with the child is on recognition and acceptance of angry

feelings and of the fact that the targets of anger are also the objects of positive feelings. As the child experiences the security
of firm limits and reestablishes positive feelings toward others,
self-starvation decreases and he or she becomes more able to
give and receive affection.

TREATMENT RESULTS: The outcome of several more years
of therapy was that Gerry began to make friends and to develop
a tentative interest in boys.

COMMENTARY: This article illustrates well the fact that adjustment and adjustment problems are often the result of cumulative success and failure in earlier developmental periods. The
girl whose case was discussed was not just someone stressed by
the onset of adolescence. She was a child with a long-standing
pattern of manipulating others through illness, one who had
missed a great deal of school and quite possibly had learning
problems, and one who had never learned how to express feelings effectively. In fact, early detection and treatment of any of
these other problems might have averted the anorexic crisis.
    As with other crisis situations, for example, suicide at-
tempts, anorexia nervosa requires two phases of treatment, one
to deal with the crisis and the other to improve long-term adjustment. We would, however, disagree with Rollins and Blackwell that the second phase should necessarily be insight oriented.
In the case presented, there was clear evidence of continued
need for specific therapies directed toward improving family interaction patterns and alleviating other social skills deficits.

SOURCE: Rollins, N., and Blackwell, A. "The Treatment of
    Anorexia Nervosa in Children and Adolescents: Stage 1."
    Journal of Child Psychology and Psychiatry, 1968, *9*, 81-91.

Operant Conditioning and Anorexia Nervosa

AUTHORS: P. E. Garfinkle, S. A. Kline, and H. C. Stancer

PRECIS: The use of individualized reinforcers to promote weight gain for five hospitalized female anorexia nervosa patients

INTRODUCTION: It is a well-established principle in psychology that to increase the frequency of any response, one should follow it with positive consequences. Garfinkle, Kline, and Stancer sought to extend the application of this principle to include weight gains in anorexia nervosa patients.

CASE HISTORY: Five girls were treated, all of whom had experienced weight loss greater than 25 percent of body weight. They all showed an aversion to food and consciously restricted their food intake. None of them was medically ill, but all experienced amenorrhea as a consequence of excessive weight loss.

Case 3 is typical of those presented: This was a seventeen-year-old girl who had for reasons unknown developed an avoidance of solid foods. Her weight had dropped precipitously and she was amenorrheic. Ward staff observed that this girl was anxious to socialize with friends off the ward and was interested in occupational therapy. After unsuccessful attempts to promote weight gain through traditional psychotherapy and through chemotherapy, it was decided to use her preferred activities contingently as reinforcers for weight gain. Off-ward socializing and occupational therapy were made contingent upon daily weight gains of at least 0.15 kg, and weekend passes were made contingent upon weekly weight gains of at least 1 kg.

TREATMENT METHOD: Treatment consisted of a number of specific steps, each involving patient participation. The hospital dietician consulted with each patient about diet and then formulated a three thousand calorie diet, taking into account patient food preferences. On the basis of patient interviews and staff observation of patient activities, a system of rewards was developed. Goals were set on minimum daily and weekly weight gains necessary to restore normal weight, and a verbal contract that tied weight gains to specific rewards was negotiated with each patient. Throughout these proceedings it was made clear to patients that the responsibility for eating and for weight gain rested with them and not with hospital staff.

TREATMENT RESULTS: Treatment led to dramatic weight gains for all five patients. In Case 3, cited above, a weight gain of 8.6 kg in six weeks resulted in a transfer to outpatient treatment. After discharge from the hospital, the patient was seen weekly for individual and family therapy sessions. At the end of nine months, weight gains made during the hospital stay were being maintained.

COMMENTARY: This method clearly places responsibility for weight gain on the patient; so power struggles with those in authority are reduced. When necessary, the reinforcement procedures used can be combined with other forms of treatment to produce a stronger or more lasting effect. In the case presented, individual and family treatment sessions after discharge probably helped to stabilize weight gains that had been achieved while in the hospital. Had there been a stronger avoidance reaction connected with eating solid foods, desensitization might have been a necessary prerequisite to the operant treatment.

SOURCE: Garfinkle, P. E., Kline, S. A., and Stancer, H. C. "Treatment of Anorexia Nervosa Using Operant Conditioning Techniques." *The Journal of Nervous and Mental Disease,* 1973, *157,* 428-433.

Anorexia Nervosa and Desensitization

AUTHOR: E. A. Hallsten

PRECIS: Brief treatment of anorexia nervosa through desensitization of fear of gaining weight

INTRODUCTION: If the excessive dieting of anorexia nervosa is prompted by a fear of becoming fat, then it ought to be possible to eliminate excessive dieting by reducing this fear. Such a tactic would represent a real shortcut in the treatment of this complex problem.

CASE HISTORY: Ann was a twelve-year-old girl who had formerly been overweight. Prompted by peer teasing and by being called "Fatty," she designed a thousand-calorie diet that, with the addition of vitamin supplements, was approved by her pediatrician. Following the diet closely, she succeeded in losing weight and continued to lose until she was twenty-five pounds underweight. No amount of pleading on the part of her parents could dissuade her from her dieting. After having been hospitalized twice because of the threat to her physical well-being, she was referred for treatment in a psychiatric hospital. She was found to have two unrealistic fears, one a fear of storms and the other a fear of gaining weight. It was decided to make these fears the focus for treatment.

TREATMENT METHOD: Fear of storms was tackled first. Ann was trained to relax through systematic tensing and relaxing of various muscle groups throughout her body. A list of frightening situations related to storms was elicited, and these were ranked from the least to the most frightening. When Ann was completely relaxed, she was encouraged to imagine the item lowest in this hierarchy. When she was able to hold this image without anxiety, the next was introduced, and so on until the entire list had been mastered.

For the fear of gaining weight, a hierarchy was constructed

that included being called to table, being at table, eating, eating fattening foods, enjoying fattening foods, and going to stand in front of a mirror and seeing that she was gaining weight. Ann was instructed to relax and then to imagine herself in a particularly comfortable situation in her home. Items from the hierarchy were introduced one by one until she would imagine the entire sequence without anxiety.

TREATMENT RESULTS: After only one treatment session, Ann ate her entire evening meal. She continued to receive treatment twice weekly for three weeks. The hierarchy was expanded to include imagining being teased by her peers for becoming fat again. Weight gains continued. There were six more weekly sessions and Ann was discharged from the hospital, having gained more than twenty pounds. Posthospital treatment consisted of family group therapy. Follow-up five months after termination revealed good eating habits and a good readjustment to home and school.

COMMENTARY: This is an extremely simple method that, when applicable, appears to reduce treatment time and cost dramatically. A strong treatment effect was evident even before family therapy was introduced, and family sessions were used more to stabilize treatment effects than to promote weight gain. It is unlikely that this simple approach can be used in every case. Its applicability probably depends upon a number of factors, including the extent to which a specific fear influences eating behavior, the extent of family pathology, and the ease with which a therapeutic alliance can be established.

SOURCE: Hallsten, E. A. "Adolescent Anorexia Nervosa Treated by Desensitization." *Behavior Research and Therapy*, 1965, *3*, 87-91.

Management of Anorexic Symptoms in a Public School Setting

AUTHORS: R. L. Stiver and J. P. Dobbins

PRECIS: Using individualized incentives and a change in stimulus conditions to decrease anorexic symptoms

INTRODUCTION: Although it is often necessary to hospitalize young people with anorexia nervosa, it is at times possible to treat anorexic symptoms in the setting in which they arise. Stiver and Dobbins report on an unusual case involving treatment of an autistic girl in a public school setting.

CASE HISTORY: This case involved a twelve-year-old autistic girl with mild mental retardation who was enrolled in a public school program for children with severe emotional disturbance. Because the program setting had its own kitchen and dining facilities, staff had occasion for close observation of eating behavior over a two-year period. During that time, eating patterns were normal. Anorexic symptoms had subsequently developed over a period of several months. At first the girl began leaving food on her plate and making remarks about people being fat because they ate too much. Because her mother was on a diet at the time, it was felt the girl was picking up some of her views about dieting from her. Problem eating continued over the next few weeks with increased verbalization about fat and thin people and about not wanting to be fat. A brief improvement was noted when school staff decided to make access to desserts contingent upon eating the main dish for each meal. However, after about a week, the girl again began refusing to eat. She gagged on her food and reacted to eating with frequent vomiting.

TREATMENT METHOD: The treatment strategy at this point encompassed two main elements. Mother was advised to stop all comments about her own diet and to allow her daughter to eat whatever she wanted, whenever she wanted it, and at school the girl was allowed access to the cafeteria, a privilege she had often requested, on condition that she take and eat small portions of all foods being served.

TREATMENT RESULTS: Beginning with the first day of cafeteria eating, progress was noted. The girl did not refuse any foods and ate all that was given to her. Changed eating was also manifest at home. She increased food consumption and decreased food aversion. Follow-up after several months confirmed a return to normal eating habits.

COMMENTARY: Although this case represents a very special circumstance, the general principles involved in the treatment used can be applied in the treatment of most young people with anorexia nervosa. These involve separating eating from struggles for control between parent and child and providing individualized incentives for a return to normal eating. In all cases the child's physician should be involved, both to rule out physical conditions that might be causing anorexic symptoms and to monitor ongoing health status.

SOURCE: Stiver, R. L., and Dobbins, J. P. "Treatment of Atypical Anorexia Nervosa in the Public School: An Autistic Girl." *Journal of Autism and Developmental Disorders*, 1980, *10*, 67-73.

Family Group Therapy for Anorexia Nervosa

AUTHORS: P. Caille, P. Abrahamsen, C. Girolami, and B. Sorbye

PRECIS: A systems theory approach to the treatment of anorexia nervosa

INTRODUCTION: A fundamental principle in the systems theory approach is that all mental or psychosomatic illness is the result of dysfunction in a human interactional group of which the asymptomatic individual is a member. The most important group to which most people belong is the family, and family dysfunction is felt to be crucial in the development and maintenance of anorexia nervosa. The behavior of the anorexic child is seen as directing attention away from interactional problems within the family and preventing family members from having to come to terms with them. Systems theory assumes that there are strong forces supporting the status quo and that attempts to influence problem behaviors directly will be met with resistance.

CASE HISTORY: Mr. and Mrs. H. were both forty-six years old and had been married for eighteen years. Ingrid was the second oldest and the only girl among their four children. Mr. H. was a successful journalist and Mrs. H. was a housewife who had abandoned a promising career after Ingrid's birth. At about age fourteen, Ingrid suddenly stopped eating, rapidly dropping in weight from 119 to 86 pounds and interrupting her menstrual cycle. After unsuccessful inpatient therapy, the family was referred to an experimental program involving outpatient family group therapy. The course of treatment consisted of seven sessions. Each session was divided into three parts: a sixty- to ninety-minute conversation between therapists and family members, a briefer private discussion between therapists and other members of the research team who had been observing, and a final summing up for the family in which comments were made and instructions were given on how family members should relate to one another during the interval preceding the next session.

The major instruction given at the first session was for everyone to maintain their behavior just as it was. It was recognized that Ingrid was opposed to treatment, and she was encouraged to express her opposition through refusal to eat and by keeping her thoughts and feelings to herself. Mother was encouraged to continue nagging her about her failure to eat. In the first part of the second session, children and parents were seen separately. In each meeting family members were reminded of the original instructions when they spoke positively of some change in Ingrid's behavior. In the children's meeting Ingrid was told that the therapists saw her behavior as an attempt to help her family solve a problem, and she was instructed to continue it. In the parents meeting Mrs. H. defined herself as the only responsible family member, implying that her husband belonged in the other group. In the summing up, all were encouraged to continue their current behaviors, and Mr. H. was given the additional assignment of taking his wife on a surprise date each week. Much resentment was expressed regarding this assignment at the next session; and the therapists, admitting having made a mistake, gave a new assignment, to spend fifteen minutes each day in group discussion of current concerns. By the fourth session, Ingrid had clearly gained weight. Although conflict between the parents was even more obvious than before, the therapists avoided tackling this directly. Instead, they focused on a minor problem behavior of another sibling to further remove attention from Ingrid as the "sick" family member. By the fifth session, Mrs. H. was more directly expressing dissatisfaction with her husband's role in the family, and the sixth session was devoted to a discussion of termination. The final session was used to sum up family strengths and weaknesses.

TREATMENT METHOD: All family members meet as a group with male and female co-therapists. The therapists observe typical interaction patterns and attempt to understand the function of the symptom in protecting family members from unwanted change. They highlight problem behaviors but instruct those involved to maintain their behavior just as it is, thereby robbing these behaviors of rebellious significance and harnessing resistance as a force for change. The therapists give additional assignments to various family members that will indirectly interfere with typical interaction patterns. However, whenever these tasks arouse resistance, the therapists come down firmly on the side of the status quo.

TREATMENT RESULTS: After seven family treatment sessions, Ingrid no longer had any difficulty with anorexia and in fact was slightly overweight.

COMMENTARY: This brief therapy was highly effective in eliminating life threatening behavior on the part of a teenage girl. The most crucial elements appear to be providing a forum for family communication, harnessing resistance in the service of change, and interfering with usual interaction patterns. No attempt was made to understand unconscious motivations or to influence behavior by manipulation of consequences. The therapists were satisfied with removing the referral symptoms even though some additional problems remained. They communicated to the family a respect for their ability to decide about future treatment needs and an acceptance of the truth that systems need not be perfect to function effectively. This approach is not for everyone and probably requires a family unit that is relatively cohesive at the start. Working with a family in which the members were bright, articulate, and motivated to participate certainly made the therapists' task a good deal simpler than it might otherwise have been.

SOURCE: Caille, P., Abrahamsen, P., Girolami, C., and Sorbye, B. "A Systems Theory Approach to a Case of Anorexia Nervosa." *Family Process*, 1977, *16*, 455-465.

Prognosis Based on Patient Variables in Anorexia Nervosa

AUTHORS: P. E. Garfinkle, H. Moldofsky, and D. Garner

PRECIS: Long-term prognosis in the treatment of anorexia nervosa as a function of treatment and patient variables

INTRODUCTION: Reacting to criticism that the treatment of anorexia nervosa through behavior modification techniques has led to long-term adverse consequences, Garfinkle and his colleagues reviewed outcomes for a large group of patients treated with a variety of therapies. They were interested not only in how treatment modality affected outcome but also in the effects of selected patient variables.

Patient variables included age at onset of anorexia nervosa; age at the time of treatment; percentage of normal weight for age, sex, and height; number of previous hospitalizations; and presence or absense of each of the following: food fads, vomiting, bulimia (excessive eating), and laxative abuse. Presence or absence of menstrual disturbance was also noted, and all patients were rated regarding social and educational/vocational adjustment. Using a special lens that could distort photographs to make the subject look fatter or thinner than its actual size, the researchers observed the accuracy of self-perception recorded and the percentage of distortion.

TREATMENT METHOD: Patients were included in the behavior modification group if they had been treated in the hospital under a treatment plan that included the use of rewards for weight gain. Patients meeting this criteria had also received a variety of other treatments, including family therapy, individual therapy, and pharmacotherapy. Behavior modification was part of the treatment plan for 40 percent of the total group of patients studied.

TREATMENT RESULTS: The patient group included forty females and two males, each of whom had been treated anywhere from one to three years previously. Most had been in their late teens at the onset of anorexia. Global ratings of clinical condition at follow-up were based on percentage of average weight attained, eating habits, presence of menstruation, social adjustment, and educational/vocational adjustment.

Condition at follow-up was rated as excellent or much improved for 50 percent of the group. Only 12 percent failed to show any improvement or had gotten worse, but ten patients had had to be rehospitalized, and two of these readmissions had followed suicide attempts. Treatment modality seemed not to be a major factor in outcome. Number of previous hospitalizations was predictive of poor outcome, as was the presence of bulimia and vomiting. Previous educational/vocational adjustment was predictive of successful outcome. The patients whose condition was most serious tended to make poor progress, and it was primarily those who had poor outcome who required further hospitalization. The four patients with excellent outcome all tended to underestimate their body size. The one patient who succeeded in commiting suicide had greatly overestimated her body size.

COMMENTARY: As is usual in studies of this type, behavior modification did not produce any greater or less effect than other therapies on a global outcome measure. Patients treated with a behavior modification approach did gain weight rapidly, but like those receiving other treatments, they continued to have additional problems that required long-term management through individual and family therapy and in some cases pharmacotherapy. The fact that there is a large number of patients who continue to have problems long after treatment underscores the importance of a long-term, continuous relationship in the treatment of this condition. The occurrence of suicide attempts and rehospitalizations should alert the therapist to the need for special precautions in follow-up. Because bulimia and vomiting are significantly related to negative outcome, it might be beneficial to apply behavior modification strategies directly to these behaviors. Techniques for dealing with bulimia and vomiting are detailed in the next section of this chapter and in other volumes of this series. Sections of *Therapies for Children with Psychosomatic Disorders* are particularly relevant.

SOURCE: Garfinkle, P. E., Moldofsky, H., and Garner, D. "Prognosis in Anorexia Nervosa as Influenced by Clinical Features, Treatment and Self Perception." *CMA Journal*, 1977, *117*, 1041-1045.

Additional Readings

Garner, D. M., Garfinkel, P. E., Stancer, H. C., and Moldofsky, H. "Body Image Disturbances in Anorexia Nervosa and Obesity." *Psychosomatic Medicine,* 1976, *38,* 327-336.

It has frequently been stated that people with eating disturbances, both anorexia nervosa and obesity, have inaccurate perceptions of their body size. This study confirms a tendency on the part of some obese and anorexic young women to overestimate body size; however, on the average, both these groups were more accurate than normal controls who in fact underestimated body size. Important findings on personality measures were that patients with anorexia nervosa scored high on introversion and that obese patients scored high on external locus of control. Also, anorexic patients who overestimated their weight tended to score higher on neuroticism than those who did not.

Munford, P. R. "Haloperidol and Contingency Management in a Case of Anorexia Nervosa." *Journal of Behavior Therapy and Experimental Psychiatry,* 1980, *11,* 67-71.

Munford demonstrates the application of a single subject research design in evaluating specific effects of multicomponent treatment of a seventeen-year-old anorexic girl. Making free time away from the hospital unit contingent upon daily and weekly weight gains appeared to accelerate weight gains and to maintain them once they had occurred. Factors beyond the control of the researcher obscured the effects of drug treatment. After discharge the girl was seen in individual psychotherapy and her parents were seen in marital therapy. The threat of rehospitalization appeared to be a factor in long-term maintenance of acceptable weight.

Piazza, E., Piazza, N., and Rollins, N. "Anorexia Nervosa: Controversial Aspects of Therapy." *Comprehensive Psychiatry,* 1980, *21,* 177-189.

Anorexia nervosa is seen as involving many levels of dysfunction. The effects of genetic predispositions, intrauterine and birth trauma, failure to master previous developmental tasks, intrapsychic conflicts, and distorted family structure and interaction are all considered in formulating the treatment plan. The treatment program is an attempt to address these problems comprehensively. Although the initial focus is on increasing weight and normalizing eating patterns, the focus soon shifts to social rehabilitation through activity groups and involvement with a special assigned nurse or childcare worker. All patients are involved in individual psychotherapy, and psychoactive drugs are prescribed for the small percentage who need them. Other family members are treated individually, in family sessions, and in weekly parents' group meetings.

Vomiting

Vomiting can result from a variety of physical causes, including illness, overeating, difficulty in swallowing, and motion sickness. It may also occur as a response to anxiety, tension, or stress. Once physical illness has been ruled out, the design of appropriate treatment depends upon a knowledge of precipitating stimuli and reinforcing consequences. When there is an obvious precipitating stimulus, some form of desensitization may be the treatment of choice; and when vomiting is maintained by desirable consequences, withdrawal of reinforcement along with reinforcement of alternative behavior is probably the optimal strategy. Punishment through such means as electric shock can be effective and should be seriously considered in situations in which there is an immediate threat to health. These strategies can all be used separately or in combination. Possible physical causes should be carefully explored by a physician before a psychological explanation is accepted.

Treatment of Vomiting Associated
with Motion Sickness

AUTHOR: D. G. Saunders

PRECIS: The use of relaxation and desensitization techniques in overcoming vomiting resulting from motion sickness

INTRODUCTION: Vomiting has a variety of causes, and even though they are primarily physiological, the possibility always exists that the consequences of vomiting may influence its rate of occurrence or that responses to related stimuli may aggravate the problem. Saunders hypothesized that because of nausea and vomiting, his client had learned to be anxious about riding in cars and buses and that this anxiety increased the likelihood that he would actually get sick while traveling. He helped the client to overcome the problem through the use of a variety of relaxation techniques.

CASE HISTORY: The client was a thirteen-year-old boy with a problem of motion sickness dating back to the age of six months. Since that time he had become sick and vomited while riding in a car or bus about four or five times each year. He avoided riding to school on the school bus and avoided some automobile trips for fear he would become ill. Occasionally, trips had to be cut short when he did become car sick.

TREATMENT METHOD: The boy learned muscle relaxation through a method involving alternately tensing and relaxing various muscles and muscle groups. Deep-breathing exercises were also part of the training. The boy was then taught to take a deep breath and tense his stomach muscles, following this with exhaling and relaxing, whenever he approached a motor vehicle in which he was about to ride. After relaxing for thirty seconds, he repeated this exercise, and he repeated it twice again after sitting down in the vehicle. Finally, he was taught to relax while imagining progressively more anxiety-arousing scenes of traveling by car and bus and experiencing motion sickness.

TREATMENT RESULTS: Vomiting had occurred one week prior to his coming for treatment, and nausea had occurred once during the pretreatment assessment period. Subsequently, there were no instances of either vomiting or nausea during the four months of treatment or during a nineteen-month follow-up period.

COMMENTARY: When anxiety plays a part in inducing vomiting, relaxation methods are likely to be important in treatment. This case points the way toward appropriate treatment, though it is not exactly clear which elements of the method described produced the desired effect. Further refinements could shorten the time required to overcome this problem. Systematic reinforcement of mastery of the problem and its associated anxieties would likely enhance the treatment effect. It might be necessary to devote specific attention to reinforcing certain behaviors, such as riding in the school bus; and attractive alternatives, such as getting a ride to school with a parent, should certainly not be provided.

SOURCE: Saunders, D. G. "A Case of Motion Sickness Treated by Systematic Desensitization and in Vivo Relaxation." *Journal of Behavior Therapy and Experimental Psychiatry*, 1976, 7, 381-382.

A Problem with Swallowing Pills

AUTHOR: G. O. Sallows

PRECIS: Treatment of a swallowing problem through repeated practice with gradually increasing task difficulty

INTRODUCTION: Often when a particular stimulus leads to a problem response, the problem can be eliminated by presenting the stimulus in small doses that are gradually increased as the client gets used to them. Sallows demonstrates how this principle was applied in eliminating gagging as a response to pill taking.

CASE HISTORY: The client was a sixteen-year-old girl with a disease of the blood. Treatment involved taking large numbers of pills each day. However, attempts to take the pills led to gagging and vomiting. The girl had a long history of difficulty in swallowing pills, and as a younger child had always taken pills crushed and mixed with food. But it was not possible to do this with all the pills necessary for treatment of this illness.

TREATMENT METHOD: It was explained to the girl that the best way to overcome the problem was to learn to take small pills first and gradually work up to larger ones. Practice was carried out with candies of various sizes and shapes rather than with actual pills. The therapist demonstrated swallowing increasingly large pieces and then asked the girl to do the same. He praised her for her efforts even when she didn't succeed. There were ten treatment sessions with several swallowing trials in each session. One to four candies were swallowed in each trial. Any time a new combination of sizes was involved, the therapist demonstrated first. Whenever the girl could not swallow the candies in three or four swallows, candies for the next trial were crushed into smaller pieces. Between sessions, there was a daily homework assignment of swallowing four small candies.

TREATMENT RESULTS: In ten sessions the girl progressed from requiring an average of more than 20 swallows per trial to requiring an average of 1.13 swallows per trial. After the sixth treatment session, she began experiencing success with actual pill taking at home. Follow-up contacts were made at five months, two years, and four years. She continued to be able to take several pills at once in one or two swallows.

COMMENTARY: This simple treatment was quite effective in

overcoming a long-standing problem habit. There was no attempt at coercion, but rather the girl was helped to gain control
over her own response. Whenever she encountered difficulty,
the demand was decreased so that success became more likely.
Such an approach has wide applicability and can even be applied to a variety of formal learning tasks that might present difficulty for some adolescents.

SOURCE: Sallows, G. O. "Behavioral Treatment of Swallowing
Difficulty." *Journal of Behavior Therapy and Experimental
Psychiatry,* 1980, *11,* 45-47.

Additional Readings

Alford, G. S., Blanchard, E. B., and Buckley, T. M. "Treatment
of Hysterical Vomiting by Modification of Social Contingencies: A Case Study." *Journal of Behavior Therapy and Experimental Psychiatry,* 1972, *3,* 209-212.

A seventeen-year-old girl with a ten-year history of vomiting after every meal was successfully treated through a behavioral approach that relied mainly on withdrawal of attention and
social isolation whenever vomiting occurred. In the first phase
of treatment, the girl was given five regularly scheduled meals
each day in her hospital room. She was attended by two staff
members, who got up and left the room each time she vomited.
Once vomiting was under control, the girl was shown graphi-
cally how social contingencies affected her behavior. To promote generalization to eating that occurred in the patient dining area, other patients were asked to respond like the therapists
to any vomiting that occurred in their presence, and an arrangement was made for the patient to spend thirty minutes in a
time-out room after any incident of vomiting. No further incidents occurred in the hospital, and during a seven-month follow-
up period, the patient vomited only once.

Ingersoll, B., and Curry, F. "Rapid Treatment of Persistent Vomiting in a 14 Year Old Female by Shaping and Time Out." *Journal of Behavior Therapy and Experimental Psychiatry,* 1977, *8,* 305-307.

A fourteen-year-old girl was treated for persistent vomiting of twenty-seven days duration. Treatment involved the systematic application of positive consequences for food retention and negative consequences for vomiting. The plan was to provide specific amounts of food at regular intervals and gradually to change from liquid to solid and increase the intervals and amount of food eaten. Each minute of food retention earned points as well as money. Points could be exchanged for opportunities to watch television and to visit other patients. Attention, praise, special activities, and food reinforcers were all available after longer periods of food retention. Negative consequences for vomiting were to involve periods of time-out, either sitting in the corner or being sent to bed. After the first treatment session, vomiting ceased. The next day the patient requested normal foods, and she was quickly returned to a regular diet. The reinforcement program was maintained throughout the next several days until she was discharged. There were no recurrences of vomiting during a one-year follow-up period.

Linden, W. "Multi-Component Behavior Therapy in a Case of Compulsive Binge-Eating Followed by Vomiting." *Journal of Behavior Therapy and Experimental Psychiatry,* 1980, *11,* 297-300.

Linden reports on a twenty-year-old female of normal weight who for four years had engaged in daily episodes of binge eating (three thousand to five thousand calories at a sitting) followed by vomiting. Initial history taking revealed that at one point she had been concerned about excess weight. She had subsequently become anorexic and still later had developed the pattern of dieting plus binge eating with which she presented for treatment. Treatment consisted of the following components:

1. Addition of an evening snack of high caloric "forbid-

den foods" to her daily intake of dietary food, such that total calories were sufficient for weight maintenance without weight gain

2. Continuous self-monitoring and self-recording of food intake

3. Family support of dieting through buying less problem food, providing a special storage place for diet foods, and bringing the late night snack to her room so that stimulation to overindulge would be reduced

4. Reinforcement of an alternative behavior (yoga exercises) as a response to hunger cues occurring outside of planned eating times

5. Assertiveness training directed toward increasing social involvement and decreasing feelings of loneliness that had served as a trigger for binge eating

Treatment was effective in virtually eliminating binge eating.

@©@©@©@©@©@©@©@©@©@©@©@©@©@©@©@©@©@©

Enuresis

Enuresis is a common childhood problem for which incidence declines throughout the developmental years. No more than 3 percent of adolescents are enuretic, but this still represents a large number of cases, and many of these young people have low self-esteem and impaired family and peer relationships as a result of their enuresis. Enuresis may be due to organic causes or it may have a functional basis. It is referred to as "primary" if successful toilet training has never taken place and "secondary" if continence has previously been achieved and maintained for an extended period of time. There may be a genetic predisposition for both primary and secondary functional enuresis, and both may involve faulty training in the preschool years as well. Secondary enuresis usually has its onset in the preschool years, and some personal or environmental trauma frequently precedes onset. Family moves, parental separation, hospitalization, and illness or death of a family member have all been implicated. Once organic causes have been ruled out, treatment for enuresis is largely a matter of training or retraining of bladder function. This may involve increasing bladder capacity and sensitivity to full bladder cues, or it may be a matter of increasing incentives for self-control. Occasionally, specific anxieties may have to be eliminated through systematic desensitization, and in cases of secondary enuresis, there are probably times when exploration of feelings concerning the precipitating event can expand self-knowledge in a way that is beneficial to the patient.

@©@©@©@©@©@©@©@©@©@©@©@©@©@©@©@©@©@©

Positive Reinforcement for
Bladder Control

AUTHOR: K. Popler

PRECIS: Elimination of enuresis through token reinforcement of nonenuretic behavior

INTRODUCTION: A simple, painless method for treating a variety of problem behaviors is systematically to reward competing behaviors. Popler extends this method to the treatment of enuresis in a teenage boy.

CASE HISTORY: David was a fourteen-year-old boy who had never successfully achieved nighttime bladder control. He was also a poor student and had few friends. The first visit to the therapist's office was used to elicit background information from David and his family and to provide instructions regarding record keeping. This was to be David's responsibility, with the parents serving as supervisors and consultants. David and his parents were asked to return in two months, at which point the record was reviewed and instructions were given for earning rewards. David returned for half-hour weekly meetings at which he received coupons for dry nights during the previous week. Fifteen coupons could be redeemed for five dollars. This requirement was raised to twenty and then to thirty-five as David experienced greater success.

TREATMENT METHOD: The first step in treatment is to establish a method for keeping a record of wet and dry nights and to determine the rate of wetting over a baseline period. The therapist then begins rewarding staying dry by dispensing coupons on a weekly basis for each dry night during that week. He or she also maintains a progress chart that the child can see at each office visit. Coupons are redeemable for money, and the number of coupons necessary for a specific monetary reward is gradually increased as success becomes more frequent.

TREATMENT RESULTS: Enuresis was eliminated after twenty-eight weeks, and control was still in effect at six-month follow-up. Schoolwork and peer relations were also reported to be improved.

COMMENTARY: This method requires minimal parent involvement and so has inherent appeal in the treatment of adolescents. It is somewhat costly in terms of therapist time, but the time investments are spread out over a fairly long period. The therapist could probably be replaced by a paraprofessional. The fact that monetary rewards are involved probably reduces drop-out rate, but parents and child should be aware of time requirements so that they don't become discouraged and leave treatment prematurely. Treatment effects might be speeded up by combining this method with nighttime waking. The family should also be given a choice regarding more intensive methods that might take effect more rapidly.

SOURCE: Popler, K. "Token Reinforcement in the Treatment of Enuresis: A Case Study and Six Month Follow-Up." *Journal of Behavior Therapy and Experimental Psychiatry*, 1976, 7, 83-84.

Conditioning Treatment of Enuresis

AUTHOR: D. J. Brooksbank

PRECIS: The use of an enuresis alarm as an aid in conditioning nighttime bladder control

INTRODUCTION: The causes of enuresis are not always clear, though it has been suggested that there is a genetic predisposition. Psychological stress sometimes interrupts previously established bladder control, and faulty training may be present independently or in combination with other causes. Occasionally, enuresis results from urinary tract infection or other organic determinants. Except when the causes are organic, enuresis can generally be treated by systematic training or retraining, regardless of specific cause. Brooksbank reports good success with adolescents using an "enuresis alarm." He also offers suggestions for preventing relapse once treatment has been successful.

TREATMENT METHOD: A complete history regarding toilet training and toileting problems is the first step in treatment. Also appropriate physical examination and urinalysis are performed to rule out an organic basis. Base rate data are collected for two weeks, during which time parents are asked not to restrict fluids or engage in nighttime waking. Only those children with a rate of wetting of 50 percent or more are accepted into the program.

Treatment involves the use of an enuresis alarm, a device placed on the child's bed that activates a bell or buzzer when the child urinates in the bed. All families who agree to participate are given a careful demonstration of its use. They are told that when the alarm goes off, one of the parents must make certain that the child wakes up and carries out previously agreed upon routines for completing urination and for changing bed clothes. Children are seen briefly every two weeks, at which time they must bring an up-to-date record of wet and dry nights. Nightly routines are reviewed in detail and praise is given for following routines and for dry nights. Once routines are well established, the interval between treatment sessions is increased. When the child has succeeded in remaining dry for fourteen consecutive nights, a change in treatment is introduced to strengthen bladder control. He or she is at that point encouraged to consume extra fluids before going to bed. Except in cases where excessive flooding of the bed indicates inadequate functional bladder capacity, this is continued until the criterion of fourteen dry nights is again achieved, at which point treatment is terminated.

TREATMENT RESULTS: Of the total of seventeen cases who accepted and completed treatment, all gained nighttime bladder control. There were three relapses, but two regained control after another course of treatment.

COMMENTARY: This approach to treatment of adolescent enuretics is quite efficient, taking only about three hours of professional time over an average five-month course of treatment. Brooksbank alludes to equipment problems, which require occasional phone contact outside of normal treatment appointments, and he mentions that an alarm booster is necessary for some children who are exceptionally heavy sleepers, but otherwise treatment seems straightforward and uncomplicated. The length of time required for the total course of treatment may discourage some families from participating, but those who do participate appear to have excellent success.

SOURCE: Brooksbank, D. J. "The Conditioning Treatment of Bed-Wetting in Secondary School Aged Children." *Journal of Adolescence,* 1979, *2,* 239-244.

Brief Intensive Behavioral Treatment of Enuresis

AUTHORS: N. H. Azrin and P. M. Thienes

PRECIS: A combination of behavioral methods applied during a one-day training period with continued daily supervision provided by parents

INTRODUCTION: The incidence of enuresis is about 3 percent among fourteen-year-olds. Neither psychotherapy nor chemotherapy has been particularly effective in alleviating this problem. Bell and pad (enuresis alarm) conditioning methods have achieved an impressive 80 to 90 percent success rate among those completing treatment, but relatively high dropout rates are a problem with this method. Contributing factors include length of time required for treatment, parental annoyance at being awakened in the middle of the night, and problems with equipment malfunctioning. Azrin and Thienes sought to develop a treatment approach that would achieve results more rapidly and would eliminate the need for a bell and pad apparatus.

TREATMENT METHOD: Training is carried out during one long afternoon and evening session. It begins with a discussion of why the child and parents are distressed by bed wetting and which other relatives and friends are also concerned and goes on to include a discussion of the rewards the child might earn by staying dry. Children are encouraged to drink large quantities of their favorite beverage and are reminded to do this at fifteen-minute intervals. At half-hour intervals, they are asked to go into the bathroom and attempt to urinate. When a child feels that he is about to urinate, he is told to hold back and is praised for his success in doing so. When he feels he cannot hold back much longer, he is told to lie on his bed in a darkened room pretending to be asleep and to concentrate on the full bladder feelings, describing them aloud. He is asked to rehearse mentally what he will do at night when he experiences similar sensations and to carry out this plan by getting up and urinating in the toilet.

One hour before bedtime the child is made to describe the cleaning up activities that will be necessary if he has an accident and to practice them twenty times. He also practices twenty times the nighttime responses that will prevent wetting, that is, waking up, going into the bathroom, and urinating. During this practice his parents remind him of the rewards to be earned by staying dry and express their confidence in him. He is encouraged to continue drinking water during practice so that urination might actually occur. He is occasionally asked to feel the dry sheets and to comment on their dryness.

During the night the child is awakened hourly for the first four or five hours after going to sleep and is encouraged to go into the bathroom and urinate. Hs ie praised for his attempt even if he does not succeed and is given another drink before going back to sleep. Children who do not want to go to the bathroom are wakened sufficiently to sit on the edge of the bed and make eye contact. If they then indicate that they can hold their urine, they are praised, given another drink, and allowed to return to sleep (fluids are not given after 11 P.M.). If the child is wet at any of the hourly wakings or if he is wet when parents check his bed in the morning, he is reprimanded and required to change his pajamas, put wet sheets in a hamper, and make up the bed with dry sheets. He is also required to practice twenty times waking up, going to the bathroom, and urinating; and he is told that he will have a half hour of similar practice that night before going to bed.

Parent follow-up involves continued nighttime waking, along with appropriate practice and reinforcement for success. On the first night parents awaken the child to toilet at midnight or one o'clock. If he is dry, his waking time for the next night is moved back a half an hour. A clock face drawing near his bed demonstrates progress and reminds parents of the waking hour for the next night. When he reaches the point when waking is scheduled for just one hour after bedtime, nighttime waking is discontinued.

In the morning, beds are checked half an hour before scheduled waking. If the bed is wet, the child is awakened, asked to clean up, and required to engage in half an hour of practice of waking and going to the bathroom. He is also told that he will have to practice for a half an hour that night. Children who sleep through the night without wetting are praised for their success and told they will have a half hour extra play that night because practice will not be necessary. Praise is provided several other times during the day, and visitors and concerned relatives are informed of the child's success. The therapist is also kept informed of progress. A progress chart is conspicuously displayed, and agreed upon rewards are provided at progress milestones negotiated during the first evening of training.

TREATMENT RESULTS: Nighttime accidents were decreased

from 90 percent to 25 percent after only one day of training and were down to 10 percent by one month for the fifty children participating in this project. All children who completed training (92 percent of those who signed up) ultimately achieved a criterion of fourteen consecutive dry nights. Occasional relapses were quickly overcome by briefly reinstating treatment.

COMMENTARY: This intensive training program has a low dropout rate and a high success rate. It involves a full day of therapist time as well as very active participation by parents and children, but it brings rapid success. There seems to be no question that the vast majority of children can be successfully treated for enuresis. The choice appears to be between highly successful intensive methods and those that are less demanding initially but will probably take longer to implement and are not always so successful.

SOURCE: Azrin, N. H., and Thienes, P. M. "Rapid Elimination of Enuresis by Intensive Learning Without a Conditioning Apparatus." *Behavior Therapy,* 1978, *9,* 342-354.

Additional Readings

Fritz, G. K., and Anders, T. F. "Enuresis: The Clinical Application of an Etiologically Based Classification System." *Child Psychiatry and Human Development,* 1979, *10,* 103-113.

After reviewing research studies on the etiology of enuresis, Fritz and Anders developed a classification system that includes various subcategories of organic and functional enuresis. In a clinical study involving 116 enuretic children between the ages of four and fourteen, they attempted unsuccessfully to validate this classification system. There were, however, significant findings regarding secondary enuresis (onset after initially successful toilet training). There was a significant correlation be-

tween the presence of secondary enuresis and early commence-
ment of toilet training. Onset of secondary enuresis was primarily in the preschool years and frequently associated with
personal or environmental trauma, such as a family move or a
separation between parents. In many cases, encopresis and
nightmares were also present.

Singh, R., Phillips, D., and Fischer, S. "The Treatment of Enuresis by Progressively Earlier Waking." *Journal of Behavior
Therapy and Experimental Psychiatry*, 1976, 7, 277-278.

A thirteen-year-old girl with a seven-year history of enuresis was successfully treated using nighttime waking. In three
years of family therapy, no observable progress had been made
in controlling enuresis. Bladder retention exercises had also
been unsuccessful. Because it was known that urination usually
occurred at least two hours after bedtime, the girl was instructed to set an alarm to wake herself after two hours so that
she could go to the toilet. After seven dry nights, the time was
moved up to ninety minutes after bedtime, and then sixty,
forty-five, and thirty minutes as she achieved continued success.
Mother was told that her daughter should clean the bed sheets
if an accident occurred, and the girl was told that she would get
a new bed after six months without wetting. During an eight-
month follow-up period after treatment was terminated, there
were no instances of bedwetting.

Stedman, J. M. "An Extension of the Kimmel Treatment Method for Enuresis to an Adolescent: A Case Report." *Journal of
Behavior Therapy and Experimental Psychiatry*, 1972, 3,
307-309.

Stedman reports on the case of a thirteen-year-old girl who
was taught a self-control procedure for overcoming enuresis.
She was given the rationale that to overcome nighttime accidents, she needed to become more sensitive to bladder distention cues. A week of self-monitoring revealed a daytime pattern
of frequent urinaton to weak cues. The girl was then instructed
to record strength of cues hourly and to hold urination thirty
minutes beyond the onset of strong bladder distention cues.
This led to an initial reduction in the frequency of urination

during the day, to increased nighttime waking during urination, and ultimately to the elimination of bedwetting.

Taylor, D. W. "Treatment of Excessive Frequency of Urination by Desensitization." *Journal of Behavior Therapy and Experimental Psychiatry*, 1972, *3*, 311-313.

Taylor reports on the case of a fifteen-year-old girl who complained of excessive frequency of urination. Urinary urgency seemed to be associated with school-related anxieties. Hierarchies of anxiety-arousing scenes were constructed in relation to the themes of "riding in a school bus," "being in school buildings and classrooms," and "actively participating in classroom activities." The girl was given training in muscle relaxation and then practiced relaxing while imagining progressively more anxiety-arousing scenes in the three hierarchies. After ten treatment sessions, excessive urinary urgency was eliminated and frequency of urination was normal. Therapy continued for five more sessions, which were devoted to discussion of family problems. There had been no recurrence of urinary problems at four-month follow-up.

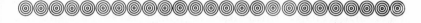

Insomnia

Inability to sleep at night generally results from tension and worry, though there may be a central nervous system predisposition to this disorder. At times, a physical illness is the initial cause of sleep disturbance, which is subsequently maintained by parental attention. With some young people, specific fears (fear of death or fear of separation from parents) may interfere with the ability to fall asleep. With others, resistance to going to bed has been conditioned by parents who send their children to bed when they have misbehaved. Treatment is usually straightforward, involving relaxation training, interruption of worry, deconditioning of specific anxieties, and rearrangement of reinforcement contingencies. Sometimes insomnia is only the most visible manifestation of more serious individual or family problems, in which case more comprehensive treatment may be needed.

A Multimodal Approach
to Insomnia

AUTHORS: K. R. Mitchell and R. G. White

PRECIS: Eliminating the sources of insomnia through the use of self-control procedures

INTRODUCTION: Difficulties in falling asleep at night can be caused by physical and mental tension or by worry and intrusive thoughts. The control of these sources of sleep disturbance may require multiple therapeutic interventions. Mitchell and White explore the cumulative effects of several self-control procedures in alleviating sleeping problems.

TREATMENT METHOD: Progressive muscle relaxation involves learning to control tension in various muscles throughout the body by deliberate tensing and relaxing. Mitchell and White provided four relaxation training sessions over a two-week period. Clients receiving this treatment were instructed to practice muscle relaxation three times a day for the next three weeks and also to focus on reducing presleep tension and intrusive thoughts. In mental relaxation training, clients are trained to visualize themselves in a variety or relaxing activities. Training and practice for those receiving the treatment involved the same amount of time as progressive muscle relaxation. Cognitive control techniques include such activities as self-commands to stop unpleasant thoughts, deliberate use of time-out from worry, and replacing irrational thoughts with rational ones. Cognitive training sessions were carried out after relaxation training. These sessions occurred once a week for three weeks, followed by two weeks of daily practice.

TREATMENT RESULTS: Thirteen males ranging in age from nineteen to twenty-eight participated in treatment. All had long-standing problems in falling asleep, and none could get to sleep at night in less than one hour. Throughout treatment, they kept records on presleep tension, intrusive thoughts, time to sleep onset, and sleep satisfaction. All treatments produced significant improvements on each of these measures, and the cumulative effect of all three was one of markedly reduced tension and intrusive thoughts and greatly increased sleep satisfaction. Time between going to bed and falling asleep was reduced on the average about 80 percent.

COMMENTARY: This highly effective approach vigorously attacks the various sources of insomnia. The amount of time actually spent in treatment is small considering the magnitude of the effect. Not only is the insomnia alleviated, but clients are given new skills they can use in eliminating a variety of problems.

SOURCE: Mitchell, K. R., and White, R. G. "Self Management of Severe Pre-Dormital Insomnia." *Journal of Behavior Therapy and Experimental Psychiatry*, 1977, *8*, 57-63.

Relaxation Training Plus Reduction in Parental Attention for Treatment of Insomnia

AUTHOR: D. R. Anderson

PRECIS: Therapy for insomnia involving new coping skills for the patient and changed response to the problem on the part of his parent

INTRODUCTION: Sleep disturbance stimulated by internal tension or excitement may be maintained by parental attention. Effective treatment then requires not only the learning of relaxation skills but also a change in how parents respond to their child when he or she is having difficulty sleeping.

CASE HISTORY: The client was a thirteen-year-old boy who

had been having difficulty sleeping for four months. Because he generally experienced tension and anxiety throughout the evening before going to bed, his mother had gotten into the habit of sitting up with him until quite late. When he finally did go to bed, he was often unable to fall asleep for two or three hours. During the night, he sometimes came to his parents' bedroom, and his mother would go with him to the living room and stay until he was ready to go back to bed, sometimes for as long as an hour.

TREATMENT METHOD: He was taught to control muscle tension through relaxation exercises in three one-hour sessions. He was instructed to carry out these exercises before going to bed and at any time he woke up during the night. His mother was told to withdraw attention gradually from his sleeping problem. The first week she was to go to bed at her regular time even if he was still up; and if he came to her bedroom, she was to go with him to the living room for only a brief time and then return to bed. In the second week, if he came to her bedroom, she was to get up and go to the bathroom, but avoid interacting with him. In the third and subsequent weeks, she was to stay in bed and send him back to his room.

TREATMENT RESULTS: The frequency of sleep disturbance was greatly diminished after only one week of treatment. By the eighth week of treatment, the patient was no longer having difficulty falling asleep. Restless behavior before going to bed and visits to his parents' bedroom during the night had also been eliminated.

COMMENTARY: Although the circumstances that precipitated insomnia were apparently never discovered, it was possible to eliminate this problem by giving the patient new coping skills and directing his mother to alter the consequences she provided for his behavior. Had she been unable to modify her own behavior so easily, it would have been necessary to explore further the ways her behavior was being maintained and to work more systematically at parent behavior change. It would not be unusual for a parent to engage in this kind of inappropriate relationship with a child in order to avoid their own problems in a marital relationship. In such a case, marital therapy might also be needed. As it was, however, the problem was quickly eliminated through short-term treatment involving only mother and child.

SOURCE: Anderson, D. R. "Treatment of Insomnia in a 13 Year Old Boy by Relaxation Training and Reduction of Parental Attention." *Journal of Behavior Therapy and Experimental Psychiatry*, 1979, *10*, 263-265.

Tics

Tics are involuntary, recurrent muscle movements. They may involve eye blinks, facial twitches, and larger movements of head, torso, or limbs. They also involve involuntary utterance of words or sounds. Tic disorders may be transient or chronic. Gilles De La Tourette Syndrome is a special category of disorder involving both involuntary movements and utterance of obscenities. It is unclear whether there are actually several discrete tic disorders or all tic symptoms are manifestations of the same underlying pathology. Tic occurrence seems to wax and wane as a function of developmental stage, environmental circumstances, and specific ongoing activities. Drug treatment is not generally recommended, though with patients having Gilles De La Tourette Syndrome, treatment with the drug Haloperidol has frequently been reported to be successful. Even when drug treatment is effective, however, it may have to be discontinued because of unwanted side effects. Behavioral strategies have the advantage of having no such side effects. Those reported to be effective include self-monitoring, massed practice, punishment, and manipulation of social consequences. Because cures are often claimed after relatively brief follow-up periods, it is difficult to determine whether reported effects represent complete cures, temporary amelioration of symptoms, or fluctuations in disease course having no relationship at all to treatment intervention. Thorough assessment under a variety of circumstances and over a prolonged period of time is an important part of the management of tic disorders.

A Multicomponent Treatment
for Tics

AUTHOR: M. Tophoff

PRECIS: The successful use of a multicomponent behavioral strategy for the treatment of Gilles de la Tourette Syndrome in a patient for whom drug treatment had produced negative side effects

INTRODUCTION: Gilles de la Tourette Syndrome is a psychophysiological disorder characterized by facial tics and other unwanted motor movements and by the involuntary utterance of sounds, including obscenities. Pharmacological treatment of this disorder with the drug Haloperidol has been relatively successful, though there are some children for whom medication is not effective and others who develop neurological symptoms, like parkinsonism, as side effects of drug treatment. There has also been some success in treating Tourette Syndrome with behavioral techniques. Tophoff describes the application of a multimodal behavioral approach to the case of a child for whom treatment with Haloperidol at low dose levels had caused drowsiness and parkinsonism.

CASE HISTORY: The patient was a thirteen-year-old boy whose symptoms included head jerking, echolalia, and the involuntary utterance of obscene words. He also frequently uttered the verbal tic "eh" in a very loud voice and was unable to desist from a habit of sticking his finger in his mouth. Treatment with Haloperidol had been ineffective in doses ranging from 0.2 mg to 0.9 mg. The only effects of the treatment were those negative side effects previously noted. Not only was drug treatment contraindicated, but neither supportive psychotherapy nor relaxation training had led to symptom relief.

TREATMENT METHOD: A decision was made to use a behavior modification strategy and to focus on the verbal tic "eh" and a particular obscene word. The major treatment intervention was massed practice (voluntary repetition of the unwanted habits over long periods of time). During twice weekly, hour-long treatment sessions, each verbal response was performed voluntarily for thirty minutes. Because when they occurred outside the treatment situation these responses were often preceded by feelings of tension, the patient was also instructed to use his previously acquired relaxation skills whenever he began to feel tense. His parents were instructed to ignore symptom behaviors rather than attempting to stop them, and they were also instructed to encourage and reward self-assertive behavior.

TREATMENT RESULTS: Treatment led to a sharp decrease in the focal symptoms, and by the fourteenth session, they had completely disappeared. In addition, other symptoms were eliminated without ever having been the focus of treatment. At a four-month follow-up, the client was reported to be free of tics and functioning well socially.

COMMENTARY: The combined approach employed by Top-hoff was effective over a relatively short time span in eliminating behaviors that had been distressing to the client, his family, and his friends. No attempt was made to evaluate the separate effects of the various treatment components, but it was established that relaxation training by itself was not effective.

SOURCE: Tophoff, M. "Massed Practice, Relaxation, and Assertion Training in the Treatment of Gilles De La Tourette's Syndrome." *Journal of Behavior Therapy and Experimental Psychiatry*, 1973, *4*, 71-73.

Augmenting the Effects of Massed Practice in Treatment of Tics

AUTHORS: K. N. Knepler and S. Sewall

PRECIS: Rapid elimination of an eye-blink tic using massed practice paired with noxious olfactory stimulation

INTRODUCTION: Knepler and Sewall reasoned that if massed practice of tics leads to inhibition of the tic response, then pairing practice with an unpleasant stimulus should lead to even more rapid elimination of the unwanted behavior.

TREATMENT METHOD: The client was a twenty-year-old male with a right-sided eye-blink tic he had had for four years. Treatment occurred in six sessions over an eight-day period with two days off for the weekend. On the first day of treatment, the client voluntarily practiced the eye-blink response for five one-minute periods, each separated from the next by a one-minute rest period. For the next four days this was repeated twice each day but with the addition that he took a deep sniff of smelling salts each time he performed the tic response. On the final day, he engaged in repeated one-minute practice periods without the use of smelling salts.

TREATMENT RESULTS: As treatment progressed, the client was able to produce fewer and fewer voluntary eye blinks. There was an increase in the number he could produce when the smelling salts were withdrawn on the last day of treatment, but the frequency remained well below pretreatment levels. Spontaneous eye blinks dropped from a pretreatment level of fifty-nine per hour to twenty-eight per hour and continued to drop subsequent to treatment; so at three-month follow-up, the rate was three per hour, and at six-month follow-up, it was one per hour. Both the client's work supervisor and his mother remarked on a significant decrease in tic behavior outside the treatment situation. In fact, his mother reported that it had stopped all together.

COMMENTARY: A total of only ninety minutes was spent in treatment in eliminating a well-established habit of four years duration. Although it was necessary to use aversive stimulation to achieve this effect, the client did so voluntarily, and he controlled the amount of stimulation he received. It cannot be said for certain, but it seems likely that the conditioning that occurred during treatment continued to exert an effect on tic frequency even after treatment with withdrawn.

SOURCE: Knepler, K. N., and Sewall, S. "Negative Practice Paired with Smelling Salts in the Treatment of a Tic." *Journal of Behavior Therapy and Experimental Psychiatry*, 1974, *5*, 189-192.

Medication Plus Self-Monitoring and Other Behavioral Treatments in Treatment of Tics

AUTHORS: E. J. Thomas, K. S. Abrams, and J. B. Johnson

PRECIS: The use of a combination of drug and behavioral treatments in the amelioration of tics associated with Gilles de la Tourette Syndrome

INTRODUCTION: The emergence of problem behaviors is probably almost always influenced by multiple factors. Predisposing conditions, precipitating stimuli, and behavioral consequences must all be considered in formulating a treatment plan. This seems especially true regarding the tics of Gilles de la Tourette Syndrome. The notion of predisposing neurological factors gains support from cases of successful treatment using the drug Haloperidol. However, systematic analysis of the conditions under which tics occur often suggests ways these problem habits can be successfully eliminated through behavioral techniques.

Either approach can be successful, but it is sometimes necessary to use both to achieve satisfactory symptom reduction.

CASE HISTORY: The patient was an eighteen-year-old male who had first exhibited tics at age five, a few months after beginning to attend school. Prior to attending school, he was described as "high strung" and "fussy." The first tics to emerge involved facial muscles. Later a barking sound and involuntary hand and neck muscle contractions were added, along with many minor leg and arm movements. Symptoms were much reduced during a one-year period at age thirteen when the patient was not required to attend school. After returning to school, he again exhibited serious symptoms; and by his junior year of high school, he had dropped out all together after an increase in tics made him nervous about attending. Some relief had been obtained with low doses of Haloperidol (1.5 mg twice daily), but larger doses made him drowsy and unable to function normally. At the time of referral to the hospital where he was treated, he was unemployed, had few friends, and did not go out with girls.

TREATMENT METHOD: Treatment was implemented only after a careful assessment period. Data were collected in several different situations. The first involved simply following the patient around the hospital ward and unobtrusively recording the number and kinds of tic that occurred and the situations in which they occurred. Similar data were also collected in situations outside the hospital to which the patient was deliberately exposed. These were selected because they seemed to pose problems for him. They included a cleaner's shop, a drug store, a church, the local high school, a restaurant, and the public library. The patient was also observed in his hospital room and in a hospital observation room. In the latter case, the focus was on verbal tics exclusively, and observations were carried out under four different conditions. It was discovered that the frequency was lowest when the patient was engaged in self-recording of tic occurrences.

The first target for treatment was the verbal tic. Initial intervention involved instructions to self-record all instances of this tic and to report totals to an observer at fifteen-minute intervals. When the observer could not be present, the patient recorded his own totals. Whenever rates reported were less than 0.5 per minute, the observer praised the patient. The patient was also taught relaxation skills and then learned to relax while imagining himself in each of the previously listed problem situations. The order followed in introducing these situations was from least to most tension arousing.

TREATMENT RESULTS: Self-monitoring led to almost complete elimination of the vocal tic, even before relaxation training was introduced. Manifestations of this tic were eliminated not only in the hospital, but also in the various outside settings where observations were recorded. Some additional minor vocal symptoms emerged, but these were quickly eliminated using the same method. Although the initial vocal tic seemed to respond primarily to self-monitoring, in the case of the additional vocal symptoms, it is not clear whether self-monitoring or the ability to relax in these situations had the greater effect. Involuntary neck movements were also reduced, but not completely eliminated prior to discharge.

Because of the dramatic effect of behavioral treatment on the vocal tic, drug treatment was at one point withdraw. However, increased excitability and tension along with two tic recurrences forced the therapists to conclude that both forms of treatment were necessary to maintain symptom relief.

COMMENTARY: This patient was treated during a brief stay in a hospital at some distance from his home. It was not possible to eliminate all tic behavior, but considerable relief was obtained. Although neither drug treatment nor behavioral treatment were completely effective alone, the combination eliminated a troublesome verbal tic and greatly reduced the frequency of involuntary neck movements. The relationship between tic frequency and school attendance was never fully elaborated. Separation problems at the beginning of school attendance could have been a factor; specific learning weaknesses may have made schoolwork difficult and unpleasant. It seems likely that chronic deficits in social skills prevented this young man from ever becoming successfully integrated with his school peer group. Given more time, possible problems in all these areas could have been more throughly explored, with necessary remediation provided as part of the total treatment program. Involvement of other family members in treatment could have decreased the possibility of recurrence of symptoms after hospital discharge.

SOURCE: Thomas, E. J., Abrams, K. S., and Johnson, J. B. "Self-Monitoring and Reciprocal Inhibition in the Modification of Multiple Tics of Gilles de la Tourette's Syndrome." *Journal of Behavior Therapy and Experimental Psychiatry,* 1971, *2,* 159-171.

Additional Readings

Caine, E. D., Mendelson, W. B., and Loriaux, D. L. "Neuroendocrine Effects of Haloperidol in an Adolescent with Gilles de la Tourette's Disease and Delayed Onset of Puberty." *The Journal of Nervous and Mental Disease,* 1979, *167,* 504-507.

A sixteen-year-old boy with Gilles de la Tourette Syndrome was treated with Haloperidol. Prior to beginning this treatment, he had also been evaluated for delayed onset of puberty. Administration of Haloperidol led to relief of the symptoms of Tourette syndrome, but there was concern that the drug might suppress developmental changes, which had only recently begun. Blood levels of uteinizing hormone and the hormone prolactin were significantly affected, but testicular growth and other manifestations of pubescence apparently were not. The authors caution against generalization from this single case study, pointing out that the patient was atypical with respect to endocrine status before treatment, that the endocrine effects that did occur could have subtle influences on development not detected in this study, and that monitoring for unwanted side effects would require large numbers of cases drawn from populations known to be vulnerable to the endocrine effects of this drug.

Schulman, M. "Control of Tics by Maternal Reinforcement." *Journal of Behavior Therapy and Experimental Psychiatry,* 1974, *5,* 95-96.

Schulman describes the case of a fourteen-year-old boy with a nine-year history of multiple tics. His problem had the effect of diverting attention from his artistically talented younger brother to himself. Within the context of behaviorally oriented family treatment, mother was instructed to ignore the tics. Communication between parents that had centered on the tic problem was channeled into family sessions. After an initial increase, tic frequency dropped off rapidly, but the family discontinued therapy prematurely and reverted to their old patterns of interaction within two months.

Surwillo, W., Mohammad, S., and Barrett, C. "Gilles de la Tourette Syndrome: A 20-Month Study of the Effects of Stressful Life Events and Haloperidol on Symptom Frequency." *Journal of Nervous and Mental Disease,* 1978, *166,* 812-816.

A ten-year-old boy, diagnosed as having Gilles de la Tourette Syndrome, was treated with Haloperidol. The authors report a decreased frequency of tics following the use of medication but indicate that, even while the boy continued on medication, there were fluctuations in the symptom picture that seemed to be associated with such external events as the beginning of the school semester. They also report wide variations in symptom frequency as a function of the activity in which the boy was engaged at any specific time. They caution those treating this disorder to look for environmental correlates of symptom variations before concluding that there has been a change in underlying pathology. They also recommend counseling parents regarding possible exacerbation of symptoms in stressful situations so that they do not react inappropriately when this occurs.

Self-Inflicted Physical Injury

All the problems described in this section are potentially injurious, though in some cases they are more annoying to others than they are injurious to self. Self-excoriation and hair pulling in particular may cause sores and infection. In most cases, these behaviors are habitual and engaged in without conscious intent. They do not reflect underlying psychopathology, though they may lead to disturbances in interpersonal relationships. They are frequently reinforced by anxious family members or friends who focus attention on their occurrence. Treatment is uncomplicated and requires such strategies as self-monitoring, rearrangement of reinforcement contingencies, reinforcement of alternative behaviors, and punishment.

Self-Instruction in the
Treatment of Nailbiting

AUTHORS: C. Harris and W. T. McReynolds

PRECIS: Reducing unwanted nailbiting behavior through self-monitoring and recording

INTRODUCTION: To control bad habits, one must be aware of engaging in them. One method of heightening self-awareness is systematically to record all instances of the unwanted behavior.

CASE HISTORY: Eighty-five college students, all of whom had problems with nailbiting, were given a variety of treatments, all of which were effective. The common element in all treatments was self-monitoring and recording. This involved placing a mark on a card "every time you find your finger or fingers touching your lips or teeth in the act of nailbiting." Those who at the same time verbalized the statement "Don't bite" did slightly better than those who only recorded, but the difference was not statistically significant.

COMMENTARY: The simple expedient of monitoring and recording nailbiting was effective in reducing the amount of this behavior. This tactic can undoubtedly be used in overcoming other unwanted behaviors as well. In some cases the addition of conditions like self-instruction, penalties for unwanted behavior, and rewards for alternative behaviors may also be necessary.

SOURCE: Harris, C., and McReynolds, W. T. "Semantic Cues and Response Contingencies in Self-Instructional Control." *Journal of Behavior Therapy and Experimental Psychiatry,* 1977, *8*, 15-17.

Behavioral Treatment of Self-Injurious Picking and Scratching

AUTHOR: P. R. Latimer

PRECIS: The use of contingent attention to increase appropriate behavior and decrease self-injurious picking and scratching

INTRODUCTION: Sores caused by scratching and picking at skin can become a serious medical problem. Treatment must go beyond medical management of affected area and attack directly the habits that cause the sores and lead to their infection.

CASE HISTORY: Latimer presents the case of a twelve-year-old girl with a long-standing habit of picking at her skin, which had resulted in numerous scabs and scars over her face, arms, and legs. Skin problems had begun six years previously with the eruption of boils in connection with a dog bite. Over the years, the habit of picking at sores had been maintained by considerable attention from parents and school staff. It had also become associated with specific activities, like watching TV, during which it occurred with increased frequency.

TREATMENT METHOD: Treatment was carried out over twenty-eight sessions and involved a number of interventions:

1. Adults were advised to eliminate all criticism and scolding contingent on picking at skin and poor self-grooming.
2. They were encouraged to pay attention positively to appropriate behaviors and were given role-playing practice in how to do this.
3. They were given instructions on how to alert their daughter in noncritical ways when she was engaged in picking and not aware of it.
4. The girl was instructed to engage in the incompatible behavior of pressing her thumb and forefinger together for sixty seconds whenever she became aware that she was picking.
5. Points were given for such appropriate behavior as

washing face and hands and trimming and cleaning fingernails. Points were also given for each half hour during which picking did not occur, and extra points could be earned during the periods just before sleep and just after waking because these times were particularly problematic. Points were displayed prominantly on a chart kept in the home. They could be redeemed in exchange for access to preferred activities, like watching TV or going horseback riding.

TREATMENT RESULTS: Picking at skin was completely eliminated after sixteen one-hour sessions. There was one brief relapse prior to termination, and there were a few brief relapses over the next several years of follow-up. Three-year follow-up revealed that the progress made originally had been maintained.

COMMENTARY: This case involves a simple application of the use of contingent attention and positive reinforcement to increase desirable behaviors and decrease undesirable behaviors. The girl who was treated was rather isolated from her parents. Increased opportunity for gaining parental attention was probably an important factor in treatment success. It seems likely that a good deal of supportive therapy and perhaps even specific instruction occurred, in addition to the previously described main approach to treatment.

SOURCE: P. R. Latimer, "The Behavioral Treatment of Self Excoriation in a Twelve Year Old Girl." *Journal of Behavior Therapy and Experimental Psychiatry,* 1979, *10,* 349-352.

Brief Intensive Treatment
for Hair Pulling

AUTHORS: N. H. Azrin, R. G. Nunn, and S. E. Frantz

PRECIS: Brief intensive treatment for hair pulling, involving heightened self-awareness, behavioral rehearsal, and social reinforcement

INTRODUCTION: Hair pulling is a nervous habit that primarily involves scalp hairs, eyebrows, and eyelashes. It can cause physical irritation in the affected area, and it may have social consequences in terms of rejection by people who find it annoying or repulsive. Azrin and his colleagues report on a highly effective brief treatment for this problem.

TREATMENT METHOD: As part of a larger study, nineteen people were treated with "habit reversal training." Nearly half were in their teens or early twenties. They reported an average duration of ten years for their hair pulling habits, and their pretreatment frequency of hair pulling averaged fifty-five episodes each day.

Treatment was carried out in a single office treatment session of approximately two hours duration. What follows is a description of the major treatment components:

1. Problems caused by hair pulling are reviewed.

2. The client learns a competing response involving grasping or clenching the hands.

3. Clients become sensitized to specific movements involved in the habit through self-observation using a mirror.

4. They identify movements that typically precede hair pulling.

5. They identify situations in which hair pulling frequently occurs.

6. Postural changes and deep breathing are taught as methods for overcoming tensions that might lead to hair pulling.

7. Clients practice using grasping or clenching the hands as

a response to situations or circumstances in which hair pulling might occur.

8. They also practice using these responses to interrupt hair pulling.

9. They are taught to take special care of the affected area, for example, by careful combing and brushing.

10. Clients are taught to practice the competing response in front of a mirror on a daily basis with the objective of making it as inconspicuous as possible.

11. They are taught to record on a card they carry with them all instances of hair pulling or strong compulsion to pull hair.

12. They are encouraged to seek out situations they have previously avoided because of hair pulling.

13. A friend or relative is involved in the latter part of the treatment session and is taught how to encourage elimination of the habit.

Throughout the treatment session, clients are praised for successful efforts. During the final twenty minutes, the therapist engages in casual conversation with the client, who is instructed to use the methods learned earlier in the session to prevent or interrupt any instances of hair pulling that might occur during this time. Although treatment occurred primarily during the single, long treatment session, provision was made for daily follow-up contact by phone. The frequency of these contacts was diminished as progress was noted. Within four months they were eliminated. One additional contact was made at twenty-two months to assess long-term progress.

TREATMENT RESULTS: The average incidence of hair pulling was reduced by about 99 percent after the single treatment session. This level of progress was maintained for several weeks. Over the following months there was some slippage; so average reduction was only 90 percent by four months and 87 percent by twenty-two months. All the adolescents who were treated showed complete elimination of hair pulling by four weeks, though two were not able to maintain good control over the longer follow-up periods.

COMMENTARY: Only brief treatment was necessary for most people to eliminate this troublesome habit, despite the fact that most of those treated had suffered with it for many years. In addition to the single treatment session, follow-up phone contacts were probably a very important part of treatment, serving to reinforce and extend learning that had already taken place. For some practitioners it might be necessary to make a special fee arrangement to cover such contacts; however, it appears that they can be brief and are infrequent after the first week. Provision for an extra office session was necessary for two clients. Availability of this option should be part of the total treatment plan, and for clients who appear to have serious limitations in self-control, it might be preferable to plan more than one treatment session right from the start.

SOURCE: Azrin, N. H., Nunn, R. G., and Frantz, S. E. "Treatment of Hair Pulling (Trichotillomania): A Comparative Study of Habit Reversal and Negative Practice Training." *Journal of Behavior Therapy and Experimental Psychiatry*, 1980, *11*, 13-20.

Operant Treatment for Hair Pulling

AUTHORS: C. J. Cordle and C. G. Long

PRECIS: Brief treatment of hair pulling through systematic application of positive and negative consequences

INTRODUCTION: Cordle and Long report on a treatment approach to hair pulling involving a number of self-control procedures as well as positive and negative consequences applied by the therapist. The treatment was highly effective with a twenty-five-year-old and a nineteen-year-old woman. Both were seen for weekly half hour sessions over a sixteen-week period.

TREATMENT METHOD: Treatment of the nineteen-year-old involved the following components:

1. Self-monitoring through collection of hairs pulled with weekly counting and graphing of results
2. Self-targeting with a new, lower target each time a goal was achieved
3. Use of incompatible responses like knitting and isometric exercises whenever the urge to pull hair occurred
4. Examination of a photograph showing the results of hair pulling whenever an incident of hair pulling occurred
5. Removal of head scarf and examination of scalp by a young male staff member each time a weekly target was not achieved
6. Positive reinforcement each time a weekly target was achieved
7. Gradual phasing out of the use of the head scarf as treatment progressed

Treatment was roughly equivalent for the twenty-five-year-old, though an additional aid for her was moving to the room where her husband was working each time she felt the urge to pull hair. She wore a wig rather than a scarf and removed it so her scalp could be examined by the physician whenever she failed to meet weekly goals.

TREATMENT RESULTS: For the nineteen-year-old, there was a gradual decline in the number of hairs pulled each week, from a high of 692 to a low of 0. Both clients ultimately achieved the goal of no hair pulling for four consecutive weeks. There were no relapses during a fifteen-month follow-up period.

COMMENTARY: This highly effective approach involves the straightforward application of positive and negative consequences in the control of a clearly defined habit. This is an area where such an approach is most likely to be effective.

SOURCE: Cordle, C. J., and Long, C. G. "The Use of Operant

Self-Control Procedures in the Treatment of Compulsive Hair Pulling." *Journal of Behavior Therapy and Experimental Psychiatry*, 1980, *11*, 127-130.

Additional Readings

Balaschak, B. A., and Mostofsky, D. I. "Treatment of Nocturnal Head Banging by Behavioral Contracting." *Journal of Behavior Therapy and Experimental Psychiatry*, 1980, *11*, 117-120.

A sixteen-year-old boy with a long-standing habit of nocturnal head banging was successfully treated in six treatment sessions over a thirty-week period. Head banging fluctuated with ongoing life circumstances. It was more frequent when the boy had something important to do the next day, and it diminished when he visited relatives or stayed overnight with friends. A variety of self-control procedures was instituted. Because head banging occurred only when he slept on his stomach, he was encouraged to sleep on his back and to arrange pillows in such a way that it was difficult to turn over. A bell was attached to his headboard so that he would wake early in each head-banging episode. A contract that specified he would receive a dollar for each night he did not interrupt his mother's sleep with head banging was negotiated. This was later modified so that six out of seven nights were required for a $5 reward. Treatment led to substantial long-term improvement but not complete elimination of the head-banging habit.

Rosenthal, T. L., Linehan, K. S., Kelly, J. E., Rosenthal, R. H., Theobald, D. E., and Davis, A. F. "Group Aversion by Imaginal, Vicarious and Shared Recipient Observer Shocks." *Behavior Research and Therapy*, 1978, *16*, 421-427.

Rosenthal and his colleagues used punishment with electric shock to suppress nailbiting behavior. Three punishment methods were studied under group treatment conditions. All clients were asked to role play nailbiting. Under the "hot seat" condition, a randomly selected member of the group received a shock for being about to bite or for actual contact of fingers with mouth. Under the "vicarious" condition, an experimental confederate feigned receiving shock. Under the "imaginal" condition, clients were asked to imagine receiving a shock. There were four treatment sessions over a two-week period. Within each session there were eleven conditioning trials. All clients felt that the treatment they received was effective in helping them to control nailbiting. There was a significant increase in nail length for both "hot seat" and "vicarious" methods, and the increase for "imaginal" treatment closely approached significance.

3

Interpersonal
Skills Deficits

The quality and extent of interpersonal interactions play a critical part in the identity formation process that is so prominent in adolescence. One has only to consider, for example, the importance of developments in relating to parents, other authorities, same-sex peers, and members of the opposite sex. Among many required skills are adequate verbal ability, effective listening and negotiating ability, anxiety and impulse control, and appropriate assertiveness. Lack of these is not often a prime reason for referral to a therapist. As the clinician explores the patient's problems, however, it may be observed that lack of one or more of these abilities can be a critical contributor to the referral problem.

The articles included in this chapter highlight two prominent areas of progress in treatment methods. The first is the integration of treatment of parents and children in responding to the problems of the adolescent. We have referred to the importance of this before, and many books describe the complex interrelationships of family members' problems (see S. Minuchin, *Families and Family Therapy*, Cambridge, Mass.: Harvard University Press, 1974). Family treatment also utilizes the second area of advances. This is the upsurge in methods of treatment based on learning theory models.

In making a choice of treatment approach, the behavioral conception begins with the view that many of the problems are learned maladaptive behaviors or poorly learned appropriate behaviors, with little or no environmental or familial reinforcement. Their prescription usually includes educative components, such as modeling, behavior rehearsal, and feedback by therapist or peers. Attempts can be made to see if more reward for appropriate behavior can be made available. Families, schools, and in some cases peers may assist with this. One useful method that has helped in family retraining for better communication is family contracting. Phillips and Blechman et al. provide two examples of negotiation training that can help the family learn to reach agreements themselves.

Application of skill training methods to treatment problems, narrowly focused or extensive, is a very active area of research and practice. We expect to see continuing developments in techniques based on close analysis of specific problems. One example, which has already been well investigated, is nondating. Several approaches have been developed and can be found in this chapter. Training or counseling in school or community problems may increasingly be used as preventive efforts with difficulties such as nondating or unassertiveness. These are behaviors that, if help is not received, can lead to increased or generalized problems later. The articles included in this chapter give the reader a sample of the array of new approaches currently available, and one may easily conclude that additional techniques will continue to appear.

Disturbed Relationship with Parents

With a teenager in the family, the range of parent-child conflicts is enormous. The sensitive teenager feels his or her efforts at independence are not respected and efforts at improvement are unappreciated. There is a chronic disagreement about the appropriate extent of independence that should be allowed. Conflict resolution is often inadequate and temporary. Parents have difficulty separating themselves from their children's issues. The parents' relationship and personal concerns may be likewise sharply criticized by the teenager. Separation, divorce, and remarriage may complicate problems and their solutions.

When professional help is deemed advisable, individual and family therapy have been the standard treatment modalities. The articles in this section illustrate the use of varied methods in restoring improved family functioning. Behavioral, skill development, and conflict resolution strategies are being rapidly developed at this time. These may be employed as target problems are identified. (Other procedures, used in families with antisocial teenagers, are presented in Chapter Four.)

Relieving Pressure on the Withdrawn
Adolescent in a Problem Family

AUTHORS: L. C. Scheiner and A. P. Musetto

PRECIS: Family and marital therapy to shift problem focus to relieve pressures on the adolescent

INTRODUCTION: This article illustrates special problems of the adolescent whose symptoms are especially reflective of parental dynamics. Although referral problems are formulated in terms of individual behavior difficulties, the authors emphasize the relation of these difficulties to private parental concerns. A treatment that produced many difficulties but ultimately allowed the son to improve significantly is described.

CASE HISTORY: Steve was fourteen and had recently refused to attend his parochial school, despite parental pressure. He did not participate in school or social activities and was out of place. He got anxious when asked to interact. He seemed stiff and fearful, handling interpersonal fears by staying home, close to his mother. This was not a good solution because he felt unable to meet parental expectations. He was explosive when asked to do chores at home, and his parents saw him as the cause of all their troubles. Previous evaluation, including a diagnosis of schizoid personality, confirmed them in their belief. After he swallowed iodine in a suicide attempt, they brought him for treatment.

The therapists saw the parents as badly conflicted, able to agree only that Steve was the problem. The mother, an anxious but generally competent woman, felt extremely dependent on her husband. Her anger toward him was expressed as drinking binges, threats to leave, and suicidal episodes. Usually passive at home, the father's response was to further bury himself in work, where he was successful.

TREATMENT METHOD: The interpretation was made to the parents that Steve's behavior was "negative loyalty," trying to do something for a family in distress. They were helped to examine what family problems he might be reacting to. For Steve, being bad was a means of identifying with his mother and calling for help from his father.

Steve, who insisted all the problems were his parents', soon refused to attend. Rather than press the point, the therapists took advantage of this to explore marital tensions. The therapists' objective was to support personal growth for each partner. For the wife, ways of achieving this were to return to school and to handle problems independently. For the husband, a goal was to be as interpersonally effective in sessions and at home as he was at work. He was helped to express feelings and be more active.

This couple showed a pattern of considerable acting-out behavior that resulted in a two-year-long, turbulent treatment. The therapists and the couple felt sorely tested by such episodes as the wife's leaving for several days, her serious suicide attempt, and the husband's announcement of a brief affair. However, the couple demonstrated that they still wished to stay together and overcome these crises.

TREATMENT RESULTS: They were helped to become more confident as individuals, as marital partners, and as parents. They were helped to see the importance of consistency in setting up rules for Steve, as well as consequences of breaking them.

The parents' increased involvement with each other allowed Steve the opportunity for interactions with others. Although gains were slow in coming, he was able to begin dating and to return to school (early attempts at a special program having failed). Treatment was terminated while the family members were still coping with significant problems. However, they expressed confidence at how much better they were coping with their issues.

COMMENTARY: A variety of adolescent problem behaviors signals the adolescent's inability to cope with parental over-involvement and marital discord. Stealing, school phobias, even psychotic behavior may be exhibited. The enmeshed family presents difficult issues for the adolescent and the therapists. In this case, the boy indicated he genuinely wanted a greater sense of separateness. The therapists helped the parents to tolerate this achievement and to turn to each other. The therapist may expect considerable backsliding while members seek new, alternative styles, as this article illustrates. The parents' response provides clues as to the degree of psychological independence that will be tolerated. The therapist's tolerance for frustration is likely to be repeatedly tested.

SOURCE: Scheiner, L. C., and Musetto, A. P. "Redefining the Problem: Family Therapy with a Severely Symptomatic Adolescent." *Family Therapy*, 1979, 2 (3), 195-203.

Using a One-Way Mirror Room with an Enmeshed Family

AUTHORS: R. B. Gartner, A. Bass, and S. Wolbert

PRECIS: Promoting the separation of an adolescent from involvement in parental discord

INTRODUCTION: This article addresses the difficulty in extricating an adolescent who is overly concerned about his parents' marital relationship. A teenager's expressions of anger at one parent can often be understood as speaking for the other parent, who remains generally silent. The involved child is less able to cope with his or her concerns. In some cases, such as this one, hostility reaches the point where one party refuses to speak to another. Here is a method that may help to restore more rational relating.

CASE HISTORY: Nick, fifteen, could not resolve his ambivalence about his college plans. He was excessively preoccupied with anger at his father. He had not talked to his father in a year, communicating through his mother, with whom he was on good terms. He announced he would not come to sessions if he had to sit in the same room as his father. Coming by themselves, his parents denied marital problems, but seemed to be suppressing serious conflicts. They were told that any help for Nick required his presence, and his mother promised his attendance the next week.

TREATMENT METHOD: Nick came for the next session but refused to participate in a session with his father; so it was decided to see him separately. He complained of his father's behavior, which embarrassed his mother and himself. To the therapists, Nick seemed to verbalize his usually reserved mother's resentment at her husband. His problems, isolation and depression, evoked concerns about his suicidal potential. After talking with the therapists, he agreed to sit in on a family discussion without taking part. At this point the parents began to argue and Nick felt he couldn't return.

To try to provide treatment, the therapists decided to have one therapist see the parents, with the other seated with Nick in the one-way mirror observation room. The goal was to provide Nick with the experience of a boundary between himself and his parents' discussion of problems. He could overhear them, but soon chose not to. The parents began to discuss their extensive differences and learned about the problems that Nick's concern about them was causing. Simultaneously, Nick accepted help in moving toward autonomy, discussing his involvement and subsequent guilty feelings related to his parents' relationship.

TREATMENT RESULTS: After eight sessions, the family was able to meet in a room together. As family therapy proceeded, the parents began to reduce Nick's role as marital referee and to support some of his moves toward autonomy.

COMMENTARY: Therapists need to assess the intensity of the

adolescent's current struggle with issues of separation and the obstacles to his or her further development along this dimension. The therapist may observe difficulties in parent-child relations from two related perspectives. First, with increasing psychological distance, the ways of relating are different and therefore inherently difficult. Second, if appropriate separation has not been achieved, the old ways of interacting become increasingly problematic. As changes in ways of relating occur, it can be beneficial to point out the accompanying changes in interpersonal perception that have occurred.

SOURCE: Gartner, R. B., Bass, A., and Wolbert, S. "The Use of the One-Way Mirror in Restructuring Family Boundaries." *Family Therapy*, 1979, *6* (1), 27-37.

Resolving Independence-Related Family Conflicts

AUTHORS: A. L. Robin, R. Kent, K. D. O'Leary, S. Foster, and R. Prinz

PRECIS: A conflict-resolution procedure with training in sequential problem solving

INTRODUCTION: The effort to be independent, one of the major developmental tasks of this age group, results in a myriad of clashes and misunderstandings. Parents and teenagers periodically or continually disagree on the extent of privileges. Frequently, this conflict is a major, if indirect, reason underlying referral for treatment. Robin and his co-workers present an approach aimed at helping both parties resolve independence-related disputes.

TREATMENT METHOD: The program was applied to twenty-four mother-son and twenty-four mother-daughter pairs. Baseline information was obtained from a tape of the pair discussing a fictional dispute and one of their own real disputes, each for a period of ten minutes. Four rated behavior categories were grouped as measures of problem solving: problem definition, listing of possible solutions, speculations regarding results of resolution, and talking based on an agreed-upon resolution. These four were part of a problem-solving model developed by D'Zurilla and Goldfried. One category, negative behavior, included cursing, threatening, and so forth.

A five-session therapy intervention was conducted. Each session began with a didactic review of some aspect of problem solving. Then the mother and child agreed upon a problem to present and attempted to reach a solution by negotiating the four steps in the problem-solving model. When the clients were unable to do this, the therapist assisted them to explain their own mistakes, gave his impressions, and directed role-playing possibilities. Reversed role play and therapist modeling were also used. Besides praising successful efforts, the therapist ended each session with a review of their work and possible application at home.

TREATMENT RESULTS: Both parents and children were better able to perform all four parts of the problem-solving sequence. This was true for both the fictional and genuine problems discussed. Although parents reported less lying and interruptions at home and adolescents reported better understanding of their parents, clear effects of transfer of gains to the home situation could not be demonstrated. The authors had several suggestions for users of this four-step procedure to increase generalization of effect. Practice work should be done at home. Part of therapy sessions could be used to plan family discussions. Including other family members, especially the father, might broaden support and skill with this method.

COMMENTARY: The method described here may have had limited effects, partly because of research design considerations. The authors acknowledge the pervasive difficulty of application of learning from the treatment place to the life situation. In addition to their suggestions for improvement, we feel that many families might require more than five sessions to learn the method and still more to apply it at home successfully. Additionally, we suggest that follow-up sessions, scheduled at two- or four-week intervals after the end of treatment, would help to sustain the use of the problem-solving procedure.

SOURCE: Robin, A. L., Kent, R., O'Leary, K. D., Foster, S., and Prinz, R. "An Approach to Teaching Parents and Adolescents Problem-Solving Communication Skills: A Preliminary Report." *Behavior Therapy*, 1977, *8*, 639-643.

A Whole-Family Approach to Conversation Training

AUTHOR: D. Phillips

PRECIS: Communication patterns within the family restored on a more rule-bound basis

INTRODUCTION: Extensive changes in extent and modes of communicating with parents are a predictable part of the adolescent process. New issues that divide family members may require changed ways of interacting to be resolved. Disrupted relationships, whether for brief or extended lengths of time, arise periodically. More effective communication overcomes reluctance to raise necessary issues.

CASE HISTORY: The therapist recommended "Family Council" because Ellen, thirteen, was timid and inarticulate with her parents. Original referral problems were depression, school and social difficulties, with crying spells. Although operant procedures had helped, her belief that her parents were considering divorce was a major problem. During the first council, her parents were verbose, made little eye contact, and Ellen kept her head down. Prior to the second session, she planned an agenda with the therapist, who assisted her to demonstrate some expressive strengths, asking the parents to listen, then to describe the feelings she had expressed.

TREATMENT METHOD: The communication skill known as "The Family Council" is a highly structured session with eleven rules. It is offered to families as an alternative to the usual unsuccessful interactions. The goal is better communication with reduced anxiety. Membership consists of the therapist, the parents and their adolescent, and significant others as determined in discussion. These may be siblings or baby-sitters, even surrogate parents, and may change from meeting to meeting, depending upon the goals of the session.

The first phase is the teaching and modeling of new communication patterns. The council meets for an hour, around a round table (to reduce the possibility of negative alignments). The therapist is more active at this point, introducing the first three rules at the start of Session 1. They are

1. Any issue, about oneself or one's relationship with other family members, may be raised by anyone.
2. No one may interrupt the person raising the issue.
3. Shouting is not permitted.

These and other rules are repeated when transgressed. They can also be restated by calling attention to the fact that they were followed. The other rules are introduced as they are needed:

4. "Dumping," judgmental insults and blame, is not permitted (for example, "You don't really care.").
5. Statements beginning with "I" are preferable. The therapist often restates others' comments in this more personal form.
6. Members should restate what they heard others say,

neither adding nor altering. The goal of this is to teach listening skills and call attention to the frequency of poor listening.

7. No one should be called to account afterwards for remarks made within the council. Comments may be dealt with only within the session, and infractions must be closely monitored.

8. A member can temporarily veto discussion of an issue. In this way, extremely sensitive issues can be identified and plans can be made to desensitize them by gradual introduction.

9. A member can ask another to leave for a short while. However, an important goal at that point is anxiety reduction around the sensitive topic, for freer subsequent discussion.

10. Members talk to rather than about one another. They must face each other and should try to have eye contact.

11. A one-minute limit can be enforced if someone tends to hog the floor.

There are additional learning experiences in the council. The family is instructed to hold councils at home, usually once weekly, gradually increasing to three times weekly. Members take turns as "referee" to increase awareness of the rules and how they are infringed. As family members master skills at the office council, therapist intervention lessens.

TREATMENT RESULTS: In short order, Ellen learned to speak for herself on nonanxious topics and began to be more assertive, at first with the therapist's help. The eleven rules were introduced during the next five sessions. The parents learned to listen and report accurately and found out what was troubling their daughter. Reassured they were not going to separate, she was able to raise sensitive issues such as sexual questions. Family meetings were stopped and individual sessions continued with focus on individual problems.

COMMENTARY: Council sessions may be introduced when an individual's problems resist change because of disrupted family communication. Phillips reports that this program was highly successful in five of the seven families she introduced to it. The program has been effective with highly verbal adolescents as well. The special advantage of this program is in increasing family members' relaxed interactions, probably rare during the recent past.

SOURCE: Phillips, D. "The Family Council: A Segment of Adolescent Treatment." *Journal of Behavior Therapy and Experimental Psychiatry*, 1975, *6*, 283-287.

A Conflict-Resolution Procedure for Single-Parent Families

AUTHORS: E. A. Blechman, D. H. L. Olson, and I. D. Hellman

PRECIS: Training for families in conflict management using "The Family Contract Game"

INTRODUCTION: The program is aimed at two major skills lacking in high-conflict families: problem-solving and decision-making skills. Coping skills are taught, using a game board. The goal is to develop and strengthen behaviors that will become preferable to the older, unsuccessful family discord. This article reports on use of "The Family Contract Game" with six single-parent families, but two-parent families can also use this procedure.

TREATMENT METHOD: The clients in this program answered an ad offering help for single parents in conflict with their preadolescent or adolescent children. There were six mother-child pairs, with four boys and two girls, aged eight to fifteen. Parental complaints were largely related to noncompliance in regard to school or house work, family relations, and self-care. One child was enuretic. Clinical psychology graduate students served as therapists. There were two pretreatment, five treatment, and two posttreatment sessions. The problem-oriented discussion part of each session was videotaped and rated on an interaction coding scale.

Both parents and children separately listed family problems. In pretreatment (baseline recording) sessions, four problems were chosen, two by each participant, and the mother-child pair was told to attempt their best solution in a five-minute unguided session. Two problems were considered in each pretreatment session, one chosen by the mother, the other by the child.

In each treatment session "The Family Contract Game" was played. Players chose colored markers. The "red" player chose the problem and drew up the agreement. The "blue" player was the complainee and banker. Each play of the game led to a contract. The game board had fourteen squares, each one carrying instructions to one of the players. The game had four "interaction units": selection of a problem for contracting, agreement on a better behavior, how to record and reinforce the new behavior, and the drawing up of the agreement. Successful completion of each interaction unit earned both play money and humorous bonus cards. Lack of resolution resulted in fines, repetition of the unit, and humorous "risk" cards. A fifteen-minute time limit was imposed for the unit. Each forty-minute session allowed for two games and a brief review.

Posttreatment format was identical to the pretreatment format. In this phase, families showed their gains by spending more time problem solving and less time on task-irrelevant behavior.

TREATMENT RESULTS: Families learned the game skills quickly, making rapid changes the first treatment session but not thereafter. The game had acted as a strong control over behavior, supporting resolution and reversing a tendency by both sides to complain more than to collaborate. Informal report suggested that there was generalization in these families, with behavior change at home believed due to the contracts.

COMMENTARY: The obvious strength of the game is in its reward of effective collaboration, without permitting interference by problems of authority issues. The game format is an excellent choice to manage conflict. It is likely to appeal more to the younger than to the older adolescent. We suggest that the game can be used in two-parent families, with the teenager having games alternately with one parent and then with the other. However, all parties must be concerned to avoid issues of splitting parents by making an agreement with one parent that the other would not accept.

SOURCE: Blechman, E. A., Olson, D. H. L., and Hellman, I. D. "Stimulus Control over Family Problem-Solving Behavior: The Family Contract Game." *Behavior Therapy*, 1976, *7*, 686-692.

Teaching the Teenager to Increase Supportive Parental Behavior

AUTHOR: A. S. Fedoravicius

PRECIS: Use of shaping procedures by the adolescent to deal with parental unresponsiveness

INTRODUCTION: This article addresses the problem of little or no follow-through on treatment plans on the part of parents. Parents may help clarify the problem, but resist changing their own patterns to help their child. Shaping is a method of changing or bringing out a desired but currently infrequent behavior. The feature of this program is the plan made to revise parents' responses so that they are better able to assist with their son's problems.

CASE HISTORY: The parents of a sixteen-year-old boy brought him for help because of a variety of problems. They reported that he stole from them and their other children, was doing poorly in school, with frequent truancy, lied, and was disobedient. The parents had unsuccessfully attempted to deal with him by physical means, monetary and other restrictions, and a prior attempt to get professional help.

The teenager described his parents as excessively demanding, carping, critical, and given to frequent lecturing. The therapist's first hypothesis was that the parents directed most of their attention to their son's unacceptable behavior and little to requested behavior. The parents' survey of their own behavior confirmed this; they showed no attention to requested behavior, which made up, in their observations, 30 percent of the boy's behavior.

TREATMENT METHOD: The first plan was to get the parents to pay more attention to appropriate behavior and less to undesirable behavior. When three weeks of attempting this did not result in any change in parental behavior, a second strategy was developed. The son received counseling on getting his parents to pay attention to what they said they wanted. He was to express thanks or make some appropriate remark after being helped. He was to begin gradually, doing this only twice a day at first. This was because of concern that his parents might view sudden changes with mistrust and increase their negative behavior. The son was recommended to respond to their critical remarks with silence. There was no discussion of whether obeying the parents would be helpful.

TREATMENT RESULTS: The son, who was seen weekly to review the program, reported no problems in finding parental behaviors to reinforce with various means of appreciation. He even asked them for help, thereby obtaining additional responses he could reinforce. After two weeks of this strategy, more frequent positive interactions and fewer, less intense arguments with his parents were reported. But he complained of getting more criticism and lectures. Instructions were to keep on being silent in the face of these. Progress continued, in the form of fewer disruptions or restrictions, fewer lectures, and a generally improved relationship with his parents. They in turn reported their son had stopped stealing and lying and was more involved around the house. Termination was after twelve sessions with the boy. Follow-up meetings at one, three, and nine months showed the improved relationship had been maintained, even in the face of occasional episodes of petty theft or defiance.

COMMENTARY: The crucial importance of obtaining the parents' help is shown here in an unusual fashion. This youngster was motivated to improve relations with his parents, and only after this happened did his antisocial behavior decrease. The procedure was acceptable to the youngster, among other reasons, because he was not preoccupied with separation and independence issues so typical of this age group. It may be more difficult to use this approach when independence is a major issue. It might be offered, in these cases, as a way of learning to keep parents off one's back, to reduce their criticism, and to escape a fight you don't want to have. The advantage of improved relations with parents may or may not be an attractive selling point.

SOURCE: Fedoravicius, A. S. "The Patient as Shaper of Required Parental Behavior: A Case Study." *Journal of Behavior Therapy and Experimental Psychiatry*, 1973, *4*, 395-396.

Improving Communications in Adoptive Families

AUTHORS: R. Pannor and E. A. Nerlove

PRECIS: Exploration and alleviation of family problems considered related to adoption

INTRODUCTION: The authors describe how special needs of adoptive families were served by discussion groups. Several families presented problems that seemed more complicated because the adolescent children presenting the problems are adopted. Pannor and Nerlove observe that adopting parents are somewhat older when beginning their families than nonadopting parents. They may feel unsure in what ways their development and troubles as parents are different. There seems to be much more anxiety in these parents when parenting crises occur. Feelings about background factors that led to adoption, such as infertility, still seem influential in current family dynamics. For the children, the fact of adoption may complicate the search for identity, with increased fantasy about the identity and motivation of their biological parents.

TREATMENT METHOD: To deal with a community need, group sessions with eight families requesting services were arranged. There were eight weekly separate sessions for parents, four sessions for adolescents only, one joint session, and a summation session for parents.

Goals for the parents' group were an accepting atmosphere for free expression of long-standing and recent concerns, exploration of how their children expressed curiosity about their bioparents, and how they felt about this interest. Talking to other adoptive parents with common problems was reasssuring, producing new ways of seeing old problems. Group members learned that the search for bioparents did not automatically undermine the strength of the relationship with the adoptive parents. Adoptive parents' role as the real, psychological parents was not erased or denied by their children's search for information about their biological origins. Such a search did not necessarily weaken the adoptive relationship, and adoptive parents could safely separate themselves from the search.

Goals for the adolescent group were to learn that many of their problems were not unique to them as individuals or as adopted children and to utilize a private place to permit expression of what being adopted meant to them. They often felt uneasy wanting to raise this topic with their parents. In the group they were able to reveal fantasies and strong feelings about both sets of parents. Several themes evoked intense involvement. The adopted children were not able to be satisfied with being told why they were surrendered for adoption. They maintained an attitude of being rejected. Fantasies and questions about biological parents' characteristics and motives for giving up their children were actively considered. Another issue was pregnancy prevention. Part of this discussion included whether a teenage mother should raise her own baby. The implications of this issue were clear to the group, which discussed it with some difficulty.

TREATMENT RESULTS: At the summation session, the parents expressed relief and appreciation about several changes. Tension stemming from adoption-related issues had receded. The children had begun to reveal private fantasies about their bioparents and spoke of emotionally upsetting topics, which surprised the parents. The children's changed behavior and improved family relationships were also noted.

COMMENTARY: Many community agencies may wish to offer services for groups of adoptive parents. The issues described in this article may also help the clinician dealing with the individual or the adoptive family. The adolescent in individual treatment may benefit when the fantasies about parents are explored and separated from whatever realistic adjustment issues are present. Parents can be counseled about the emotional strength of their relationship and the similarity or differences of their problems to those of nonadoptive parents. They can also develop more effective responses to their children's demands. An important goal is to reduce adolescents' anxiety and guilt about their anger and increasing separation from the people who made a home for them.

SOURCE: Pannor, R., and Nerlove, E. A. "Fostering Understanding Between Adolescents and Adoptive Parents Through Group Experiences." *Child Welfare*, 1977, *56*(8), 537-545.

Integrating Stepfathers into
Troubled Families

AUTHOR: M. H. Mowatt

PRECIS: Exploring special problems of stepfather-adolescent relationships in reconstituted families

INTRODUCTION: With increasing divorce rates and remarriage, there are more children and adolescents with stepparents, having to learn to live together. There are twice as many stepfathers as stepmothers. The uncertain role of stepfather, with conflicting expectations and values, can breed confusion on all sides. Several such families were asking for help with their children's (aged ten to seventeen) behavior difficulties. They were formed into a therapy group.

TREATMENT METHOD: In addition to remarriage, another major change had occurred: These mothers had been working but were now at home. Peer discussion soon revealed how anxious all were at the possibility of making mistakes in childrearing.

The stepfathers lacked initiative in the discussion. The problem arose about how far to go in taking a fatherly role. The men had become attracted to the women, not their offspring. They wondered how much affection to give the children and how to express it properly. They felt pushed in this area, and the wives began to wonder if they had unwittingly stimulated crises between their husbands and their children.

Support of husband's privileges and rights of discipline were examples. Wives and husbands spent inordinate amounts of time on the little, annoying frictions. The men's views on bathing, table manners, wearing shoes at home, and such would receive no support from their wives. They would then feel like outsiders. They would nevertheless be asked to effect discipline, but their wives tended to disrupt this process, feeling attacked themselves for their children's faults. Showing their conflicted loyalties, they communicated lack of support for their husbands.

This was an opportunity for the children to express lack of respect, leading to confusion about the extent of the stepfather's authority.

Some issues were unrelated to the children: remarriage was not the perfect solution to all problems. The men were castigated for not filling a "rescuer" role. The women began to see that their criticism pushed their new husbands farther from the children. Negative comparison with ex-spouses were a common form of low blow. Another major problem was undiscussed sexual wishes and disappointments.

TREATMENT RESULTS: This group was warmly supported by the parents, who found an accepting peer group. They became better able to present their expectations and accept the less pleasant side of their relations with the youngsters. In general, the adults' improved relationships were followed by progress observed in the children.

COMMENTARY: The author speculates about these men who chose to marry women with children. Issues of inadequate mothering for these men were noted, as well as poor relations with their own fathers and siblings. Such marriages may have represented opportunities to repair or compensate for prior emotional deprivations. For the adolescent, arrival of a replacement parent with different expectations of family functioning complicates an already problematic struggle. It may draw him defensively closer to his mother while he is simultaneously attempting greater separation. Groups such as this provide rich opportunities for exploration of past and present family crises. The follow-up Mowatt reported suggests that this can be a successful intervention, often requiring little or no further individual therapy.

SOURCE: Mowatt, M. H. "Group Psychotheapy for Stepfathers and Their Wives." *Psychotherapy: Theory, Research and Practice,* 1972, *9*(4), 328-331.

Additional Reading

Sugar, M. "Group Therapy for Pubescent Boys with Absent Fathers." *Journal of the American Academy of Child Psychiatry*, 1967, 6, 478-496.

This article reports on the group treatment of twenty boys referred for school and behavior problems. All had absent or deceased fathers. The boys were between eleven and a half and thirteen years of age. The group was never larger than ten boys at a time. Art and other play materials were available. Limit setting was continually required for most of the boys, who showed hostile dependency. Providing snacks helped reduce some aggressive behavior.

Defenses against fears of abandonment emerged when the therapist announced the cancellation of the fourth session. As the boys became more involved, discussion of sexual themes emerged, with some homosexual anxieties being visible to the therapist. The boys expressed pleasure when, after several months, their mothers began their own discussion group. Several sessions later they began to discuss feelings about their fathers. Themes of identification with fathers, mothers destroying fathers, ideal father behavior, and anger at desertion by others emerged. Use of play material decreased as the boys interacted more verbally. In general their adjustment improved, with the therapist noting that they were engaged in more growth-oriented and typical adolescent activities.

Socialization and Communication Deficits

The problems in this section include poor ability in interacting with peers and authorities and inadequate verbal skills, such as holding a conversation, listening, and expressing oneself effectively. These lacks contribute to complication of problems, may make treatment more difficult, and should be considered important targets for intervention. Recent innovations in this area have stemmed from assumptions that these skills have been inadequately learned, poorly reinforced by the environment, or both. Treatment programs aim to train better responses and assume that these changes will lead to more positive gains and eventually become self-reinforcing. Some of these programs have utilized a group training model while in the development phase. Peer-group training can be a valuable therapeutic experience. However, many of the techniques used to help these youngsters learn can be adapted for individual or family situations. These include modeling, rehearsal, role playing, role switching, and structured feedback. Help with these problems can be offered as part of a more broad psychotherapy, as a separate treatment process, or as a preventive intervention for youngsters at risk.

Group Training for
Socialization Deficits

AUTHOR: J. J. Pease

PRECIS: A sequential program providing training with a range of psychosocial problems

INTRODUCTION: Applying social skills training to help adolescents is a recent development. Developers of training programs are faced with helping people who have had little incentive or opportunity to learn and use these coping skills. Parents' poor communication skills and their problems with other family members or with authorities are some examples of factors in their children's later social development problems. In training programs designed for a socially underskilled population, extensive thought must be given to group design and curriculum. Pease gives a clear example of the procedures used in putting together a program.

TREATMENT METHOD: Six children, aged ten and a half to fourteen, of both sexes, comprised the group. Criteria for selection were interpersonal problems in the area of friendlessness, poor expression of thoughts or feelings, and little social awareness or shyness. Psychiatric diagnosis was not used to select or screen out (though delusional and hallucinating children were not included). The leaders hoped for a variety of strengths and weaknesses in a group.

The pregroup phase began with a screening interview and an orientation to the family on potential benefits of the group. Attention here was directed toward examining how better relationships would help all with problems. The group design and need for a commitment to attend were mentioned. Video and audiotape equipment to be used were shown to the family.

The training phase employed both educational material and a group dynamics focus. The educational focus was on both verbal (loudness, pitch, and inflections) and nonverbal (posture, facial expressions, and gestures) elements. Nonverbal elements proved to be a good introduction to group discussion. Help was needed for people to find the words to express what they saw, to give feedback to others. Examination and imitation of small behaviors and of common social rituals was done, raising discussion of the use of social conventions. Video feedback was helpful in members' learning about the impressions they gave.

Techniques and conventions in conversation were reviewed next. Topics included taking turns in talking, taking up another's topic or handing over a topic, and awareness of the listener. Mirroring (repeating back) and having to reply to another with an exploratory question were some techniques used. Answers were reviewed with audiotape feedback. Members practiced in pairs.

Finally, social behavior was rehearsed. Conversations were practiced outside of context; then complete situations were rehearsed. Practicing and role playing took up the first half of a session, followed by video feedback. Therapists made sure that praise was given for good use of skills and that correction was low key.

As for group dynamics, a major element at the outset was group cohesiveness or team building, using firm leadership and structure, with group games and support of weaker members. Therapists made clear that part of the objective was to have some fun as well. During the group's middle phase, acceptance of self-disclosure and exploration of challenges to leadership were major themes. During the final sessions, separating from valued people and reviewing what was learned were the major issues. Extra work was necessary for those group members who had absent or deceased parents.

TREATMENT RESULTS: The program was especially effective with anxious, shy, and socially awkward younger adolescents, according to Pease. The outgoing, less anxious youngsters who had followed available maladaptive adult models were observed to be less responsive. This group may have been less motivated, having achieved some success through deviance.

COMMENTARY: Pease's work is especially noteworthy for the

exposition that different skills are best learned at different group stages. This combined didactic and group dynamics approach avoids the simplistic assumption, now large discredited, that a group experience leads to gains in desired skills. Instead, the knowledge of group issues arising at each stage was used to explore different themes at each point. We feel that an extremely important, though often neglected, step is to plan for postgroup maintenance of gains by follow-up groups. Perhaps this is more important for the children making fewer gains. Counseling of parents on supporting new behaviors is advised. Another step to help children hold on to gains is to help them become assistants, if there are subsequent groups.

SOURCE: Pease, J. J. "A Social Skills Training Group for Early Adolescents." *Journal of Adolescence,* 1979, 2, 229-238.

<hr>

A Social Skills Training Curriculum for Younger Adolescents

AUTHORS: W. R. Lindsay, R. S. Symons, and T. Sweet

PRECIS: Content and guidelines of a well-evaluated program

INTRODUCTION: The program described here has been modified over several trials to respond to special needs of younger adolescents. It is a lengthier program than many others. This article features a summary of the issues in setting up the group, ten broad topics, and a structured format.

TREATMENT METHOD: The program has served socially unstable adolescents, referred mostly from psychiatric and child guidance facilities. Major problems are isolation, shyness and poor social interaction, and aggression. Ninety percent of the youngsters have completed this voluntary program. The speculation is that the youngsters see the group as practical and the feedback they receive as being given in positive ways.

A predetermined format is necessary. It relieves the awkward, shy teenager of having to take initiative at the start of training. The beginning of each session is a free-play period, to help relationship building, which is necessary for later communication exercises.

Staff observation of the free-play activity yields information on the youngsters' functioning that the adolescents themselves cannot provide. Further information on their problems is sought from adults close to the teenagers. The teens themselves do not describe their problems well.

A prepackaged topics list is not used, nor is there a time limit on discussions of a single topic. One issue may be discussed for weeks until all parties feel it has been sufficiently covered. Two-and-a-half-hour weekly groups are held in a room with games available and snacks provided at the start. Coffee is available throughout the entire session. The first three meetings have free play as the primary activity but also allow teaching the rules of interacting, observing, and giving feedback in a positive way. The session format is then introduced: a free-play period, an hour of work on skills, a role-play time, discussion, and review. As skills are acquired in the program, the youngsters are advised to try them in the free-play time.

The topics that have proven to be worthwhile, in the authors' opinion, are (1) *nonverbal communication,* including appearance (modeling, role playing, and rehearsal are used), (2) *nonverbal aspects of speech,* such as tone (clarity and length of speech are discussed and role played), (3) *verbal aspects of speech,* including questioning, giving personal information, giving opinions, and expressing interest (discussion and role playing are used), (4) *starting conversations* (approaches used are modeling and role playing), (5) *joining conversation groups* (approaching, seeking cues to join in, and becoming involved in the general talk are discussed), (6) *assertion skills* (this is the longest session, often lasting eight to ten weeks, and includes both influencing and influence-resisting responses), (7) *keeping out of trouble* (expands the issue of resistance of negative influence), (8) *dealing with authority figures* (another lengthy topic, utilizes role playing of both friendly and difficult interaction), (9) *interviewing skills* (this is intended for the older group, looking toward job searches), and (10) *heterosexual interaction* (the boys and girls role play asking for dates, making arrangements, talking, and dancing).

TREATMENT RESULTS: Evaluation showed lowered anxiety, shyness, impulsivity, and aggressiveness. A notable exception was a boy whose increased skills led to feelings of loss of control. His antisocial impulses upset him. When he got into trouble over this, he received special attention in the group.

COMMENTARY: Programs such as this are applicable to extended inpatient and residential settings as well as community program. All programs should be tailored to the needs of the client population. The fact that this program was revised several times suggests that patience and sustained effort are needed to develop a truly effective program. Some trial and error is to be expected, and openness to revision and new requests from the group is advisable.

SOURCE: Lindsay, W. R., Symons, R. S., and Sweet, T. "A Programme for Teaching Social Skills to Socially Inept Adolescents: Description and Evaluation." *Journal of Adolescence,* 1979, 2, 215-218.

Paraprofessional Guidance and Modeling for the Adolescent with Major Social Skills Problems

AUTHORS: L. M. Ascher and D. Phillips

PRECIS: Integration of behavior therapy and guided *in vivo* practice with serious disabilities

INTRODUCTION: Specific problem analysis and employment of trained guides are two special features of this program. It is adaptable for children, adolescents, and adults and is used for social as well as skill problems. Problem analysis is followed by construction of a related task hierarchy to be mastered with the guide's assistance. The guide's work is integrated with the therapy sessions, which prepare the patient for the outside training. The four case examples include work with late adolescents.

CASE HISTORY: Doris, eighteen, was resisting the program at a sheltered training workshop where she had been referred due to neurological impairment. She was quite negative, with a poor self-image, and both she and her parents were receiving help. Parental counseling included desensitization, operant principles and procedures, and assertiveness. Although this was helpful, these principles were not being used at Doris's workshop. A guide was assigned to work with her at this place, with certain tasks:

  1. To express praise for specific efforts or accomplishments
  2. To model, help rehearse, and encourage more appropriate behavior
  3. To help her form better verbal statements to peers

The guide's instructions were to respond as quickly as practicable.

TREATMENT METHOD: The patient is exposed to *in vivo* modeled behavior. The behavior models, or guides, are recruited and screened for interest in helping, clarity of communication, and assertiveness. Training for guides includes methods of positive reinforcement, rehearsal, assertiveness training, being a behavior model, and desensitization. Written material is read, discussed, and the techniques are practiced, with much use of role playing.

TREATMENT RESULTS: Doris improved in several areas, including productivity, assertiveness, and independence. She started traveling to work without help and with minimal absence. Afterwards, she found a nursery teacher aide position.

Other cases described (young adults) demonstrated help with problems such as conversing, cooking, ordering in restaurants, and preparing term papers. Although several cases had neurological problems, this technique is not restricted at all to persons with such impairments.

COMMENTARY: Use of the paraprofessional guide can assist in treatment of problems extremely resistant to change or that require extra help to effect successful transfer of training to the life situation. Overlearned maladaptive habits and problems of change in severely disturbed individuals are some situations that might be helped by this arrangement. Supervision of the guide is clearly essential. The authors do not discuss any problems of "fading," the phasing out of the guide's work. Care should be taken to avoid overdependence upon the guide and to accept the patient's efforts to go it alone when ready.

SOURCE. Ascher, L. M., and Phillips, D. "Guided Behavior Rehearsal." *Journal of Behavior Therapy and Experimental Psychiatry*, 1975, 6, 215-218.

Remediation of Deficits in Verbal Expressive Skills

AUTHORS: P. H. Davis and A. Osherson

PRECIS: Identifying and treating poor language skills in treatment assisting with a range of interpersonal problems

INTRODUCTION: A poor command of language can deprive an adolescent of the following tools: (1) a method of easily venting feelings; (2) a way of influencing people; (3) an alternative to impulsive acts; (4) a rich opportunity for human interactions; and (5) an aid to getting a perspective on one's situation and achieving insight. It also hinders the verbal aspects of therapy. Although poor verbal skills is not a common reason for treatment, this lack underlies many difficulties and could become a therapeutic target. This article reports on improvement of language problems hindering social adjustment and presenting obstacles to psychotherapy.

There are several contributors to language insufficiencies. In more traditional blue-collar families, the male role includes little discussion of feelings and little recreational reading. Language is action related, with unilateral statements, as opposed to interchanges. It is harder to learn that language can be a tool for mastery over one's affective side. The forty adolescents whose treatment is reviewed in this article had a variety of problems, but all showed a lack of language skills appropriate to their age and developmental stages.

Lack of verbal expressive skills is seen as underlying such problems as impulsive behavior, fear of speaking in class, absence of experience with abstract concepts, and frustration at not being understood. The authors clearly assume that the poor expressive levels reflect true skills deficit rather than resistance to treatment. Rather than refusing to express themselves, they are simply unable to use language to interact effectively with the environment. Lack of verbal skills may make therapy, an essentially verbal interchange, that much harder. Modifications are needed to conduct effective therapy, which may lead to better verbal skills. This can help the person to use therapy better and, more important, to function effectively in his familiar home environment. Lack of verbal skills should be identified as a treatment issue early on.

TREATMENT METHOD: Several aspects of treatment are considered. The following themes, if identified, are recommended: (1) It helps to express your feelings more clearly. This lesson can be taught in several ways. *Restating,* offering one's perception of what the adolescent is trying to say, can lead to fuller discussion of a problem. New words to describe feelings, such as powerless, lonely, restless, ashamed, and irrational, can be introduced at timely points and may later be employed by the adolescent. For example, a girl wanted her boyfriend to act differently toward her, but only when the word *tender* was presented and discussed did she know how to tell him clearly. A boy with an extreme on-and-off relationship with his girl became able to tolerate a steadier pattern after the concept of ambivalence was presented in a few sessions. (2) Transferring lessons learned from one situation to another requires special handling. Adolescents may rarely recall "similar" situations. One approach is to present hypothetical situations using real people. In the case of a patient who felt like killing a teacher who had reneged on an agreement, the therapist imagined for the patient a situation with the patient as a seven-year-old. The patient was asked to see himself as the wronged, disbelieved sibling, unable to influence the situation. Asked if that was how he felt, the adolescent agreed, and added two real examples. Examples using hypothetical people, but with the same features as the real situation, can also be presented. (3) A variety of more active techniques is advised, as opposed to waiting for associations. Some adolescents will tolerate and respond to questions well. Try to clarify and explain feelings at early stages in treatment. This may help in early engagement in treatment. Because they so rarely look at themselves, they may respond well to similar interpretations repeated many times. When the adolescent asks a question about behavior, you may assist self-searching by offering two or more possible explanations. (4) Role playing, with the adolescent taking his own part, assisted in dealing with usually repressed feelings and fantasy material. These patients had learned that to discuss anything at home was a provocation that would only bring on worse conditions. Some felt unequipped to verbally handle private feelings that would get a negative parental response. Role playing provides a safer forum for examining these private concerns. It may gradually help the patient to begin observing his own behavior while it is happening, to check himself better. Role reversal should be later in treatment.

COMMENTARY: There are a number of interesting techniques in this summary article. Some aim at developing cognitive and verbal intrapersonal skills; others are interpersonally focused. The therapist must decide at an early stage which are the primary areas of concern in the verbally deficient youngster and then choose from among these and other ways of assisting verbal competence. There is another modification not explicitly mentioned by the authors but implicit in their examples. These patients may raise many specific incidents as a way of seeking help. Whichever methods are used, it is advisable that they receive at least partial solution of the issue raised. Their concreteness makes it hard to stray too far from the direct question. Another consideration not mentioned is assisting the families to respond positively to increased verbal productions of their troubled teenagers. This important potential reinforcer for new skills can be a crucial item, especially during the first tentative stages of treatment.

SOURCE: Davis, P. H., and Osherson, A. "Modified Techniques for Therapy with Inarticulate Adolescents." *American Journal of Psychotherapy,* 1978, *32*(4), 533-543.

A Movement-Based Therapy for Inarticulate and Impulsive Adolescents

AUTHOR: R. S. Schachter

PRECIS: Structured movement games and exercises to promote awareness and subsequent verbal expression of feelings and conflicts

INTRODUCTION: Inarticulate and impulsive youngsters express their conflicts in action, which often creates additional problems for them. Activity therapies employ procedures for nonverbal expression of conflicts in a therapeutic manner. Current approaches include nondirective, psychoanalytic-interpretive, and behavioral, all using play material or games. The goal of Kinetic Psychotherapy, as described by Schachter, is the constructive expression of feelings using children's games, with active limit setting and interventions by the therapist. A primary goal, in addition to behavior change, is enhanced self-esteem.

CASE HISTORY: Gary had done poorly in a year's verbal therapy, where he had been referred for school problems such as aggression and hostile behaviors. He was in a learning disabilities day school. A physical skill development program had apparently only increased his destructiveness. In one kinetic therapy session, Gary was consistently unable to intercept a ball, being in the middle of the circle in a game called "Frustration." When his face contorted, the therapist stopped the action, asking all the adolescents what they felt at the moment. Excitement and fear were mentioned, but Gary's answer was "confused." He was able to add that he had similar feelings when reading and that he felt helpless. He then related this to arguments with his father, in which he felt like a failure. In role playing, he acted himself, then his father, and finally himself again, getting help with expressing his anger constructively. The group then returned to the ball game, where Gary's sustained effort to intercept the ball finally succeeded.

TREATMENT METHOD: The method is to create safe situations in which people usually feel moderate emotions, not easily explained away. A session usually starts with thirty minutes of activity work, after which a forty-five-minute verbally oriented therapy group is conducted. Games may evoke different emotions. An example of an anger game is a bombardment game, in which teams of youngsters throw soft sponge balls at each other. In "Freeze-Tag" the usual response when touched by someone on the other team includes frustration. Other feelings arise when one is waiting to be "unfrozen" and freed. Observing strong feelings in a youngster is a good signal for an intervention. Stopping the action, the therapist assists one or more youngsters to say what they feel. This can be followed up in the verbal session, where alternatives are explored.

The activities are closely led, and both activities and verbal interactions are monitored for hostile and other negative behaviors. The therapist identifies and limits negative interpersonal behaviors, such as baiting, scapegoating, and bullying. Otherwise therapist comments tend to be descriptive rather than interpretive.

TREATMENT RESULTS: When the games are over, the youngsters are still excited and involved with each other and able to transfer their involvement in more verbal ways, to discussing either the games or other issues.

COMMENTARY: This is a clearly explained method for younger adolescents whose poor verbal ability hinders work in other forms of therapy. It should be remembered that the author uses the kinetic exercises and activities in the service of better verbal production and emotional engagement. Although described as a group modality in this article, the technique is adaptable to individual treatment. Schachter has himself employed it in family sessions (R. S. Schachter, "Kinetic Psychotherapy in the Treatment of Families," *The Family Coordinator,* 1978, 283-288). It is not clear whether the techniques encourage regression, which could make them less suitable for older adolescents who are preoccupied with appearing grown up.

SOURCE: Schachter, R. S. "Kinetic Psychotherapy in the Treatment of Children." *American Journal of Psychotherapy*, 1974, *28*, 430-437.

Additional Readings

Chandler, M. J. "Egocentrism and Antisocial Behavior: The Assessment and Training of Social Perspective-Taking Skills." *Developmental Psychology*, 1973, *9*, 326-332.

Training of young delinquents in taking roles and perspectives of others was associated with reduced delinquency at eighteen-month follow-up. The youngsters were helped to act out skits in small groups, which were recorded. Plot and development were left to the youngsters, but there were four conditions: The stories must be realistic, nonfantastic; they must be about people their own age; everyone took a turn playing each part; and each "take" was reviewed by the group to consider how to improve it. There were ten weekly three-hour sessions. With suitable modifications, we believe role-taking training can be useful with a variety of problem populations.

Yokley, J. M., and McCarthy, B. "Multimodal Behavior Therapy: Use of Professional and Paraprofessional Resources." *Psychotherapy: Theory, Research and Practice*, 1980, *17* (1), 10-16.

An eighteen-year-old male, described as severely incompetent socially, was seen by the psychotherapist in conjunction with paraprofessional help. The "companion" was able to gather reliable data and implement *in vivo* treatment plans. One major premise was that generalization of learning was better if circumstances were similar to the original learning. A second was that diverse problems required a range of therapies: behavior, affect, sensation, imagery, cognition, interpersonal relationships, and drug treatment (the BASIC ID approach of Arnold Lazarus). Within these seven treatment categories, forty-three specific problems and procedures were detailed. The first treatment phase was aimed at establishing a modest degree of comfort and ability to exercise social skills. The second phase was to exercise these newly learned skills away from the companion. Forty-eight sessions with the psychotherapist and a hundred twenty-two hours of paraprofessional time were used. By the end of these sessions, this youngster had developed many new social and problem-solving skills. He developed a friendship and became independently active.

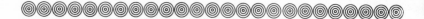

Lack of Assertiveness

Problems in appropriately holding and expressing opinions are found in many people besides psychotherapy clients. The most likely contributory factors are fears of the consequences and generalized social skill deficits. Several popular books on assertiveness have appeared, but there are still few reports of utilization of assertive training with adolescents. Helping adolescents to assert themselves effectively can result in lowered anxiety and increased confidence, assisting a more positive identity formation.

Learning to Refuse Unreasonable Requests

AUTHORS: R. M. McFall and D. B. Lillesand

PRECIS: Response practice, modeling, and coaching in a training program for assertive refusal

INTRODUCTION: Resistance of inappropriate requests is a frequent problem in the unassertive teenager. Quality of judgment often suffers under pressure by peers and groups. McFall and Lillesand have developed a procedure that may strengthen refusal responses.

TREATMENT METHOD: This procedure was developed in the laboratory with male and female undergraduates who rated themselves as unassertive, with a special difficulty in saying no. These people showed interest in receiving help for this. The training problems were taken largely from the conflict resolution inventory, a collection of validated descriptions of situations where people found refusal difficult.

In pre- and posttests, the method that seemed to produce the best gains began with a short lecture, stressing that learning and practicing effective responses in nonanxious practice situation conditions could help people be more successful in real-life stressful conditions. The individual sat alone in the room, with a tape recorder operated by an experimenter observing through a one-way window. After the narrated incident was played, the task was to practice a response *covertly*. That is, he or she was to imagine responding but say nothing aloud. The tape then played two model examples of assertive refusals (one by a male, one by a female). Then a brief discussion of the necessary elements of an effective response for this situation followed immediately. The subject then rethought his or her answer. The situation was replayed and covert responding was again requested. Over two training sessions, ten refusal scenarios were presented in this manner. Although for this group pretest and posttest refusal behavior was measured by having the subject respond aloud, during the training phase their answers were never spoken aloud.

As part of posttesting, an additional, insistent-request type was played until the person either yielded or refused a total of five times. Additional posttesting was in the form of a telephone call several days later with a persistent but spurious request for help with an envelope-stuffing task. This was to see if real-life refusal had begun to take hold.

TREATMENT RESULTS: The subjects' self-ratings of assertiveness were generally improved for this group (less positive but significant results were obtained with the group who followed the model described but responded aloud instead of covertly). In behavior ratings, posttest, and follow-up phone call performance, marked increase in ability to refuse was evident. No change in manner of speaking was observed. The authors concluded that rather than learning a new behavior repertoire, these subjects were now able to accomplish something they had known before but had not been able to do. An additional finding was that generalized assertion did not change. Apparently, knowing how to refuse did not help with positive assertion—this needed to be taught as a special skill.

COMMENTARY: This structured sequence seems adaptable for individual or group therapy utilization. Refusal behavior is an important but difficult skill for this age group, where peer pressure is often so pervasive. The utility of refusal skills in acting-out populations, as well as unassertive groups, should be explored. It might be helpful to combine this training with general assertiveness training. This might assist with development of what we might call prosocial refusal, not covered in this work. This requires specific request refusal within a generally positive interchange. We would welcome the development of such a program.

SOURCE: McFall, R. M., and Lillesand, D. B. "Behavior Rehearsal with Modeling and Coaching in Assertion Training." *Journal of Abnormal Psychology,* 1971, *77,* 313-323.

Treating Abused, Nonassertive Females

AUTHORS: J. E. Meyers-Abell and M. A. Jansen

PRECIS: Assertive training and counseling to modify a passive-aggressive response style in an abused adolescent wife

INTRODUCTION: Many arrivals at recently developed shelters for battered women present as passive, helpless, and prone to feeling guilty. This contrasts with a frequently cited picture of the abused wife as intrusive and dominant. The authors present a case of a late adolescent female treated in their assertive therapy program after being beaten by her husband.

CASE HISTORY: This eighteen-year-old had married after becoming pregnant four years ago and now had three children. Both partners' fathers had abused their mothers. No violence was reported until two months after marriage, when physical and verbal abuse began. Disputes concerned the husband's poor efforts at finding and keeping work, his mother's intrusiveness, and jealousy on the part of both husband and wife. She had no friends or family support. Leaving for the shelter meant, she felt, the end of love and marriage. Evaluation at entry showed mild depression (on the Beck Inventory) and a nonassertive style. However, she showed more reactive outbursts than most other arrivals at the center.

TREATMENT METHOD: The assertive program at the shelter was a two-hour, thrice-weekly, ongoing group of two to seven women. In this short-stay center, women attended from two to fifteen meetings. A therapist, structuring the meetings, had members reveal reasons for coming or current issues. Much peer support was felt as members shared new fears, explored problems, and offered solutions. Problem identification was followed by a suggestion phase and supported by role playing to assure better expressiveness. A discussion of respecting others' positions was included. Meetings closed with review of some aspect of assertiveness, such as assertion versus aggression, examining the passive-aggressive style, compromising, or requesting.

This young woman stayed at the shelter for a month, participating in ten sessions. The application of the program was shown by examination of jealousy in her marriage. Her husband disliked her attentions to anyone else, and she felt uncomfortable at his even looking at other women. She reported his fascinated observation of a woman and her response—tipping his soda into his lap. Admitting her outbursts, she stated she did not know what assertiveness was.

TREATMENT RESULTS: She learned to express her reactions to others' behavior and to make requests, avoiding timidity or excessive demands. The boundary between self-control and controlling others' behavior was extensively explored. Even after she learned the words, her anger was difficult to control. Over time, her proneness to outbursts diminished. When she left the shelter, her depression score had decreased on the Beck Inventory and assertiveness was notably increased. Follow-up at one year showed maintained freedom from depression, increased assertiveness, and several crises effectively negotiated. She had managed independent living, some less troubled time with her husband, and a separation when he resumed abusive behavior.

COMMENTARY: This program used both didactic and peer support elements to help modify responses to abuse. Several indicators of generalized improved behavior were identified, notably a period of stability and a more rapid response to her husband's renewed abusive behavior. We note that younger adolescent females, seeking the attention of boys, perhaps risk receiving similar types of maltreatment, though we have not found references to programmatic attempts to assist them. A program similar to this, available at clinics or schools, might be beneficial at earlier ages, possibly serving a preventive function.

SOURCE: Meyers-Abell, J. E., and Jansen, M. A. "Assertive Therapy for Battered Women: A Case Illustration." *Journal of Behavior Therapy and Experimental Psychiatry*, 1980, *11*, 301-305.

Additional Readings

Hedquist, F. J., and Weinhold, B. K. "Behavioral Group Counseling with Socially Anxious and Unassertive College Students." *Journal of Counseling Psychology*, 1970, *17*, 237-242.

Undergraduates were offered a problem-solving group experience led by doctoral counseling students. Behavior rehearsal was extensively used in one group. Subjects role played responses to their problem situations. The ineffective parts of their responses were identified. Performance evaluation consisted of immediate positive and negative group feedback. Behavior was rehearsed repeatedly, with occasional modeling and coaching. A second group, using social-learning theory, set four group rules: honesty in responses, responsibility for all acts and statements, helpful provision of feedback to other members, and a commitment to carry out group plans. The leaders guided problem-solving discussion, pointing out rule breaking, discouraging discussion of motivation, and pressing for action plans.

Both groups met weekly for six weeks. After three weeks, a sharp increase in assertiveness was seen in these groups, compared with controls. These differences were no longer significant after six-week follow-up. Longer training time and more consideration of application of these skills might improve treatment effects.

McFall, R. M., and Marston, A. R. "An Experimental Investigation of Behavior Rehearsal in Assertive Training." *Journal of Abnormal Psychology*, 1970, *76*, 295-303.

The technique of behavior rehearsal helped nonassertive undergraduates increase assertiveness. The rehearsal program began with an introduction to the treatment rationale and featured a presentation of six pretaped situations, four times each, for a total of twenty-four trials. After each trial, an assertive response was encouraged. The response was recorded. It was played back immediately, or the responder was given time to reflect, without feedback, on his or her performance. After expressing an opinion about the quality of the response and reviewing parameters of assertiveness (such as directness, voice quality, and ex-

pression of feelings), the next trial was presented. In a second
session, the prerecorded trial had a stimulus situation, an initial
assertive response, and a more challenging remark from the original questioner.

The results suggested that a short course of structured
practice could yield increased assertiveness within a brief period
of time. Generalization to outside situations were successful.
There was a trend (not statistically significant) for those receiving tape playback of their performance to do best, especially if
they were severely inhibited.

Dating

The common view is that one should have experience, skill, and comfort in socializing and dating by late adolescence. In reality, significant numbers of late teens feel insecure in the presence of the other sex. Many have dated rarely or not at all. What worsens the problem for these people is their assumption that these problems are rare. Recent years have witnessed the development of treatment designed for rapid elimination of dating problems. These may be treated in brief programs or as part of a wider therapy effort.

Treatment of Dating Problems
Due to Anxiety

AUTHORS: H. Arkowitz, R. Hinton, J. Perl, and W. Hamadi

PRECIS: Providing dating practice with volunteers to reduce anxiety and increase dating frequency

INTRODUCTION: The authors believe that for most nondaters, the major problem is anxiety, rather than inadequate socializing ability. They note that several explanations of infrequent dating exist, with corresponding treatment programs. These are skills deficit, conditioned anxiety, negative cognitive self-statements, and concern with physical attractiveness. Arkowitz and his co-workers believe that, even for nondaters helped in skills training programs, perhaps the major gain is reduced anxiety due to increased practice. They have developed an inexpensive program that requires little professional time and can help large numbers of clients. This article summarizes the results of several studies and efforts.

TREATMENT METHOD: Volunteers of both sexes answered a notice, indicating a wish to improve comfort and frequency of dating. At the outset, dating frequency averaged one every other month, and many had not dated. At a group meeting, several steps were taken to ensure that the program itself did not produce too much anxiety. It was emphasized that this was practice, not a dating or matching service. They were told that no attempt to find good matches between partners would be made. In fact, only minor effort was made to avoid unfortunate pairings. It was stressed that all daters would be volunteers. They gave basic information (age, address, and so forth) and any major undesired characteristics for a partner (race, height, age). Then, at weekly intervals, they received the name and phone number of an opposite-sex volunteer. No instructions were given regarding who should initiate contact, length of date, or what to do. Six such "dates" were offered.

TREATMENT RESULTS: For most volunteers, major changes were noted, including sharply increased dating frequency. More often than not, these dates were *not* with partners found by the practice project. Lessened anxiety as shown by measures taken before and after the practice dates was typically reported. One follow-up investigation reported these effects still present fifteen months later.

Practice, rather than instruction, was clearly the major factor. Use of experienced volunteer daters and of a postdate feedback sheet were unable to increase positive effects any more than the model described here.

COMMENTARY: The authors' point appears to be well supported for the anxious daters. The clinician is advised, however, to assess carefully whether this is true for the office patient who includes a poor social life among other complaints. Claims of lack of skills should be investigated carefully, and issues of social anxiety should be explored. A genuine skills problem might be approached by some of the techniques described in other articles in this section. The individual therapist may assist the anxious patient by offering counseling about the primary inhibiting effects of anxiety upon performance.

SOURCE: Arkowitz, H., Hinton, R., Perl, J. and Hamadi, W. "Treating Strategies for Dating Anxiety in College Men, Based on Real-life Practice." *The Counseling Psychologist,* 1978, 7(4), 41-46.

Direct Treatment of Anxious, Infrequent Daters

AUTHORS: L. R. Pendleton, J. L. Shelton, and S. E. Wilson

PRECIS: A multifaceted program using relaxation, skill training, and practice assignments

INTRODUCTION: College counselors find frequent complaints of inhibition or anxiety about dating or other social interactions. The authors present a treatment plan to improve social behavior. The program attacks three contributing factors to inhibited dating: anxiety, lack of skills, and the tendency to have negative self-thoughts. The plan includes the broadening of effects beyond the training phase by "homework" assignments. It was developed using university undergraduates who were infrequent and anxious daters.

TREATMENT METHOD: All sessions began with systematic relaxation training, with the aim of achieving a rapid, voluntary relaxed state. Following this, a male and a female leader would describe and model a useful skill. Among these were attending and listening, posture, and a series of increasingly complex conversational skills. In male-female pairs, students practiced and received feedback. Students were encouraged to note their doubting self-thoughts during interactions. In groups, these were read aloud and discussed, revealing how commonly people had such doubts. The group also received training in thought stopping to control these negative habits. Suddenly thinking "STOP!" in the middle of a doubt served to reduce its impact. Another exercise provided reality information: males discussed their reactions to certain things women did while the women listened, and then the women gave their views on men's behaviors, as the men listened. Both sexes reported being enlightened by this interchange.

Homework assignments were assisted by recruiting volunteer "trainers" who were self-described comfortable and frequent daters. Assignments were in two parts each week: to practice the skills learned in each session with a trainer, in or near the student center, and then with another person in another setting. Skills assigned were gradually increased in complexity and length, from a simple hello to a two-hour date.

An example of the training program was the third session. Twenty minutes of relaxation was followed by ten minutes of report on the previous homework and thoughts or doubts that might have affected performance. The new assignment, responding in conversations by associations, was presented, modeled, and reviewed to obtain additional suggested possibilities from the group, then practiced. Pairs practiced, receiving feedback. In the last part of the session, homework was assigned: three five-minute conversations with the trainer, one with another person, with negative thoughts to be noted. Relaxation was also to be practiced at least twice.

TREATMENT RESULTS: Evaluation of the total program showed significant decrease in several measures of anxiety and social fears. It was also noted that within the group, relationships were being established. These were viewed as being helpful, presumably temporary, transitional relationships.

COMMENTARY: The present program, like that of Arkowitz et al. (see previous article) answers a clearly defined therapeutic need. Although the inhibiting factors described are not a complete list of the problems associated with dating fears, they are clearly defined, with a treatment response for each one. The issue of generalization of effects is addressed, but there are no data to demonstrate that the daters' outside socialization was increased. Programs of this type should make increased efforts to obtain this information.

SOURCE: Pendleton, L. R., Shelton, J. L., and Wilson, S. E. "Social Interaction Training Using Systematic Homework." *Personnel and Guidance Journal*, 1976, *54*(9), 484-487.

Treating Social Anxiety by Desensitization

AUTHOR: H. Arkowitz

PRECIS: Presentation of desensitization as a coping skill in an anxious, minimally experienced male

INTRODUCTION: Interpersonal and heterosexual functioning were severely impaired in this late adolescent student. Multiple symptoms, including obsessional and suicidal thoughts, stemmed from his reaction to his problems with a girl. The author presents a behavioral explanation of the problem and of the treatment program.

CASE HISTORY: Anxiousness and depressive thoughts were Ted's preliminary complaints upon referral. After reporting concentration difficulties and social isolation as well, he mentioned that his relationship with his girlfriend was the greatest pressure upon him. She was his first girl. He felt possessive, jealous, and made many inappropriate demands for her attention. Their sex life was frustrating as well; Ted either lost his erection or ejaculated prematurely.

TREATMENT METHOD: Treatment was in two main parts. The first allowed for expression of feelings about his girlfriend, also reviewing his social behavior and emotional reactions. He received *in vivo* assignments to increase his activity on campus. His impulsive actions were reviewed with the aim of substituting more reasoned actions. Role playing was employed to assist this.

The second part was introduced when, after fourteen sessions, Ted ended his relationship with this girl. He was ambivalent and extremely upset about this. With the therapist's help, a goal was set to gain control over the anxiety. Desensitization procedures were employed in the following manner:

1. *Description.* Ted read a written description of the prac-

tice and theory of desensitization. A selection from Wolpe and Lazarus was recommended (J. Wolpe and A. A. Lazarus, *Behavior Therapy Techniques*, New York: Pergamon, 1966).

2. *Relaxation training.* After a training session in the therapist's office, four hours of home practice with a training tape was enough for Ted to relax effectively.

3. *Development of hierarchies.* Three lists of items in increasing order of difficulty were compiled: bothersome ruminations, anxious situations associated with his former girlfriend, and new encounters with girls.

4. *Self-managed progression* through the desensitization sequence. To support the self-control procedure, Ted worked at home, reporting to the therapist when consultation was needed. He began with five to ten minutes of relaxation, imagining a negative situation briefly, then longer if he felt no anxiety. When anxious, he stopped imagining and relaxed again. He worked up to more anxiety-provoking scenes.

On his own, Ted creatively enhanced this effort. When he found himself tensing in anticipation, he developed positive thoughts and soothing images that counteracted the tension. Ted extended generalization of his reaction to his girl's possible calls; he did this by relaxing, then having a friend dial his phone number.

TREATMENT RESULTS: Ted came to relate without depression or anxiety to many situations associated with his former girl. Ruminations also declined, and social and dating behavior resumed. He dated one girl steadily, enjoying kissing and petting without upset. He maintained these gains at follow-up and continued to respond successfully to minor crises with self-administered desensitization. Two and a half years later, he informed the therapist of his marriage.

COMMENTARY: Arkowitz stresses the often underestimated capacity of the troubled youngster to cope when anxiety is handled. (See also our previous digest of Arkowitz et al.). A notable feature of the account is the therapist's self-assigned role: consultant to the process of learning to cope. Ted was able to accept help with no report of typical adolescent resistance to advisers. It is not clear how well this would work with the rebellious youngster still heavily preoccupied with independence from adults. If these issues are prominent in treatment, it may be better to wait for a more opportune time. Also of note is the attraction of this technique to the compulsive adolescent.

SOURCE: Arkowitz, H. "Desensitization as a Self-Control Procedure: A Case Report." *Psychotherapy: Theory, Research and Practice*, 1974, *11*(2), 172-174.

Additional Readings

Curran, J. P., and Gilbert, F. S. "A Test of the Relative Effectiveness of a Systematic Desensitization Program and an Interpersonal Skills Training Program with Date Anxious Subjects." *Behavior Therapy*, 1975, *6*, 510-521.

The authors found a skill training program to be superior to anxiety reduction treatment in producing greater interpersonal dating skills (both groups showed reduced anxiety and increased dating at about the same level of gain). The skills training effort was conducted for undergraduate groups of both sexes and included (1) defining and discussing a skill and its importance; (2) viewing videotapes of poor performances of this skill, obtaining comments and suggestions, then viewing a better example; (3) rehearsal of the skill, with videotaped role playing and group feedback; and (4) weekly assignments to record the use of the discussed skill, to be reviewed in the next session. Cotherapists, a man and a woman, led eight ninety-minute sessions. Skills covered included offering and accepting compliments, asking for dates, listening skills, assertiveness, nonverbal interactions, improving appearance, dealing with silence, and handling physical intimacy. Gains made by this group were maintained at six-month follow-up.

Melnick, J. "A Comparison of Replication Techniques in the Modification of Minimal Dating Behavior." *Journal of Abnormal Psychology*, 1973, *81*(1), 51-59.

Melnick argues that replication and self-observation methods probably produce the best gains in dating behavior. From available replication, or replaying, techniques (psychodrama, simulated games, and so forth), he used a participant modeling method and vicarious conditioning, using self-reported infrequent daters. They first viewed videotapes of a heterosexual couple interacting. Several tapes, depicting increasing stages of closeness, were used in the study. Behaviors were then role played with female volunteers in front of a one-way mirror. The experimenter, behind the mirror, made additional suggestions during this phase. Videotaped performance was reviewed. Evaluation showed rated improvement on "appropriateness, masculine assertiveness," anxiety level, and overall pleasantness, with self-ratings of improved performance as well. Repeated role playing and debriefing are easily adaptable to clinical formats.

4

Antisocial Behavior

This chapter contains articles dealing with a broad range of behaviors. Some of the sections relate to specific problems, such
as aggressiveness. Others are concerned with individuals who
may exhibit many problem behaviors. There is also a wide range
of severity of behaviors in this chapter, ranging from brief episodes of running away to severe assaultive behavior. The common element is a deficiency in social or interpersonal concern,
evidenced as major inability to interact in a positive social manner. The most frequent and prominent feature of these persons
is behavior that causes psychological or physical damage to persons or property.

Attempts have been made for many years to explain the
causes of antisocial behavior. In the last century, terms like

187

"moral imbecility" were employed to suggest that there was a basic defect in the nature of such people. More recently, attention has been paid to the difficulties these youngsters have had in growing up. Psychological and sociological studies have looked at contributing factors such as family breakdown, parental abandonment, use of alcohol and drugs, the decline of morality and extent of societal permissiveness, the narcissistic, consumer-oriented culture, pressures of poverty existing in close proximity to abundance, and the continued pervasiveness of barriers to success based on ethnic background.

In has become clear, however, that explanations of problems such as delinquency using these factors are subject to many exceptions. Antisocial behavior can be found in all classes and among all ethnic groups. These explanations in addition are largely unhelpful in contributing to effective treatment planning. As with patients considered in other chapters of this volume, attention must be closely paid to aspects of the therapeutic relationship and to consideration of specific intervention practices. An additional consideration is the existence of the quality of family interaction.

It is generally acknowledged that antisocial adolescents represent a most difficult treatment group. They exhibit extreme elements of an already erratic pattern of interaction with adults. The therapist may be subjected to adoration, hate, and indifference within a short span of time. Although writers disagree on specific approaches, there is general agreement on the need for more activity and energy by the therapist than is usual in treating adults. The likelihood of the therapist's developing strong emotional countertransference reactions during the process is frequently mentioned.

Major problems in dealing with the more serious offenders arise from severe problems in family relations. Long histories of domestic strain are common, and the teenager may be estranged from the parents, who commonly feel they no longer have any influence on his or her behavior. Without the family's positive influence, a valuable resource for treatment is lost. Articles in the section on the predelinquent and early delinquent teenager show how, even in tenuous family relationships, interventions may be surprisingly fruitful in alleviating serious antisocial patterns.

Programs dealing with the antisocial adolescent frequently attempt to use effective group approaches. For reasons including family estrangement and awareness of social penalties, adolescents in these situations show a generally negative response to authorities and other adults. However, peers (who often see more fault in others than in themselves) may pressure others to see their problems and change, even while resisting help for themselves. However, as Harari's article shows, adolescents have a hard time hearing unpleasant news even from each other.

Recent developments in treatment approaches to adolescents' severely antisocial behavior rests on analysis of their behavior deficits. Verbal and communication skills deficits, inability to utilize fantasy or imagery, and low self-esteem are some examples reported by authors in this chapter. Methods to remediate these problems are constructed, often within a residential or total-treatment program. The aim is to develop a repertoire of new behaviors incompatible with former antisocial tendencies. If responses to new reinforcement conditions develop, these antisocial youngsters, it is hoped, might come to prefer these alternate responses. This body of work is growing rapidly. Reardon and Tosi and Alexander and Parsons present programs attempting to change specific inadequate behaviors in their delinquent patients. Efforts such as these require careful evaluation, including follow-up. Effective programs of this type could be especially important with these youngsters, whose response to treatment is often poor and whose cost to society for treatment, incarceration, and payment for destruction is great.

⊚◎⊚◎⊚◎⊚◎⊚◎⊚◎⊚◎⊚◎⊚◎⊚◎⊚◎⊚◎⊚◎⊚◎⊚◎⊚◎

Running Away

This behavior is usually considered an attempt to escape a home situation perceived as intolerable and unalterable. Runaway reactions vary greatly in severity; however, even the mildest category (see Orten and Soll) implies seriously impaired or absent communication with parents. Based on the adolescent's extent of antisocial involvement and the extent of home problems, help may range from effecting reunion to assisting in final separation. For a significant number of runaways, reunion with parents may be impossible.

⊚◎⊚◎⊚◎⊚◎⊚◎⊚◎⊚◎⊚◎⊚◎⊚◎⊚◎⊚◎⊚◎⊚◎⊚◎⊚◎

Classifying Runaways and
Selecting Treatment

AUTHORS: J. D. Orten and S. K. Soll

PRECIS: Selecting treatment approaches based on appraisal of problem severity

INTRODUCTION: The authors distinguish several classes of runaway problems and suggest differing responses to each. Their typology requires assessment of two factors. The first, *alienation,* seems to have increased in recent years, with greater numbers of families breaking up and poorer family and neighborhood support networks. Growing unemployment and reduced need for unskilled labor are some factors making it harder to move toward independent adulthood. Rising divorce rates suggest poor home atmospheres for increasing numbers of children and adolescents.

The second factor, *extent of prior running,* reflects the adolescent's adoption of fleeing as a possible solution to his problems. A *first-order* runaway is running for the first time and fits into one of two groups. "Walkaways" are relatively normal, do not feel powerless, and have a far from hopeless home life. They can see the flight as a learning experience and may get productive responses when they return. "Fugitives," however, are generally younger and feel more helpless, both at home and on the run.

Second-order runners are in serious conflict about whether they can or want to live at home. They accept running as a nonextreme alternative. Some express opposition through one major undesirable behavior (such as using drugs), others, by continual friction with parents.

Third-order runners, generally older, have rejected their families and become street-wise. They are not usually interested in treatment and are by now unwanted by their families. They will sometimes accept help at a runaways' shelter, but treatment requires correctional agency pressure.

TREATMENT METHODS: For "walkaways," treatment consists of effecting reunion, with family counseling to develop
alternatives to future running. Investigation of neurotic dynamics or parents' problems is probably counterproductive. For
"fugitives," prognosis is better if they connect with a special
community runaways' shelter. Counselors will need to be ener-
getically involved with the fugitive's family, which may be having major problems at this time.

The first treatment issue for second-order runners is
whether continued living at home is advisable. If not, a future
goal is friendly relations between the emancipated child and parents, discussing the issues from their separated vantage points.
If the runner stays, the family should be seen in treatment as a
unit to work out problems. The runner should be asked to bring
issues to sessions rather than to run. It may be helpful if there
are external pressures on the youngster, such as probation,
pressing him to try harder to stay.

Third-order runners resist attempts to traduce their alienated style, but may accept counseling for independent living.
Limited family contact can be made around independent living
issues, perhaps establishing links for improved relations much
later. Families may sometimes attend sessions.

COMMENTARY: Orten and Soll remind us that this specific behavior of running must be understood in family context for an
intelligent choice of treatment to be made. (Their second factor, habit strength of running, seems to us of secondary importance in comparison.) The range of interventions, from assisting
reunion to coercive intervention, follows from individual and
family assessment. Articles on treatment of runaway behavior
are few, especially in the area of "coercive" procedures (see the
introduction to this chapter).

SOURCE: Orten, J. D., and Soll, S. K. "Runaway Children and
Their Families: A Treatment Typology." *Journal of Family
Issues*, 1980, *1*(2), 249-261.

Treating Runaway Adolescents
with Overinvolved Parents

AUTHOR: G. L. Cary

PRECIS: Family and individual treatment to assist psychological separation

INTRODUCTION: The author described two cases where running away was one of the prominent symptoms. The runaways' histories suggested that running away represented a response to pressures of parental overinvolvement in their life at a time when their preoccupation was with separation. Specifically, overconcern with their increasing impulses, including issues of sexuality, resulted in an acting out response.

CASE HISTORY: Cary reported two case illustrations. A sixteen-year-old male had a history of sexual antisocial behavior. These incidents aroused the interest of his father, who would question him exhaustively, punish him, and then make up by giving him something (including a trip to a topless club). To the therapist, the boy's running and acting out was a request for effective, consistent control. This never came, and he was eventually incarcerated.

A sixteen-year-old girl, in residential treatment for a year, showed an increase in drug use and acting out, including runaway incidents and promiscuity. This increase occurred when plans for her return home were mentioned. Her running began after her visits to her divorced father became disappointing, due to his involvement with his new girlfriend. Difficulty handling her resultant sexualized feelings led her to run frequently, either to a boy her mother disliked or to casual liaisons.

TREATMENT METHOD: The author's treatment, in addition to individual sessions with the teenagers, included family therapy. Clear goals were set, both for the adolescent and for the parents. For the teenager, these included acceptance, based on increased understanding, of the internal conflict. The adolescent wished both to preserve and separate from the identification-based relationship with parents. Another goal was the shift from a narcissistic involvement, enhanced by acting out and separation, to a more mature interrelating with others based on acceptance of responsibility and commitments.

For parents, one aim was to help them understand their adolescent's parental projection, that is, how they were seen in a distorted fashion. They were asked to say *no* confidently where indicated and accept differences in views without needing to force a change. Another major issue to be resolved was the parents' separation of their own self-image from their child's. The parents' narcissism suffered inappropriately when their children acted out. Separation of self-images reduced this narcissistic intertwining. Pressure on the youngster and parents was then relieved. Each party could express differences rather than creating them by acting out.

For the teenage girl, components of the therapy process included confrontation of the acting out and ambivalent feelings, support of her attempts to discuss problems with her mother, and her conflict over independence versus maintaining family relationships. Therapy allowed her to rework issues around being controlled.

COMMENTARY: For this treatment approach to be useful, the adolescent and his or her parents must have some remaining feelings of attachment. Cary makes a point about the need for confrontation and the need for the adolescent to accept responsibility for actions taken. This is similar to others' views on the psychotherapy of the acting-out adolescent. In addition, however, the cases reported lead to the hypothesis that therapist intervention is not likely to be enough without parental willingness to assume effective control.

SOURCE: Cary, G. L. "Acting Out in Adolescence." *American Journal of Psychotherapy*, 1979, *33*, 378-390.

Psychotherapeutic Beginnings for
Impulsive Adolescents

AUTHORS: J. Weinreb and R. M. Counts

PRECIS: Building a working alliance with runaway adolescents using psychodynamic interpretation

INTRODUCTION: The authors review problems of entry into treatment with early and middle adolescents whose main problem is impulsive behavior. Some parents hope this problem is temporary and make minimal reaction. In the office, mutism, defiance, anxiety, and the wish to flee all contribute to the therapist's difficulties. These youngsters have inadequate controls over their impulsive urges and have not received protective parental restraint. The procedure described here has been used with forty impulsive adolescents, with about two thirds of these subsequently staying for treatment at least six months.

CASE HISTORY: Jean, age twelve, was brought for help after having run away four times within a month. She appeared passive, resistant, and was extremely unkempt. She answered briefly or not at all. She presented as indifferent but soon stated that home life was unhappy. Their grandmother, with whom she lived, favored her brother over her. She would not discuss herself for most of two sessions. The therapist finally asked why she was there and challenged her expressed ignorance, saying she appeared to play dumb. She agreed, adding that she did so at school. She didn't like school and this made it less likely that anything would be expected of her. Asked what she liked, she named a variety of sports activities. She agreed that these were things done mostly by boys. The interpretation offered was that she didn't like being a girl much. She agreed, citing reasons and clearly showing anger. Next session she was better dressed, talking freely of fears, including injections, and describing her earlier history. Abruptly, she mentioned a girl who dressed like a boy, claiming voice pitch was the only difference from boys. Pressed to name another difference, she retreated to playing

dumb. The second direct interpretation was that she was denying the anatomical difference and her jealousy at not having a
penis. She agreed this was why she was angry. Now the values
and advantages of being female began to be explored. Her outside behavior, including school performance and appearance,
notably improved.

Larry, sixteen, also came from divorced parents and was
a runaway. He had lived in several places and talked freely
about hating Massachusetts, his current place. Wanting to leave,
he felt held back by his mother's indecision, adding that a person should act quickly on his ideas. The first interpretation was
that Larry was afraid to wait, fearing he'd lose his chance. The
therapist added that Larry looked under pressure, perhaps wanting to run from something. Next session, Larry started by describing himself as happy-go-lucky. Soon after, the therapist remarked Larry didn't look happy to him. Larry returned to his
theme of leaving for New York, and the therapist reiterated the
theme of running from something. Larry nodded, but that was
all. The third session brought evidence that bad impulses about
his two-and-a-half-year-old sister were linked to an urge to run.
Interpretation was made but not responded to directly. Several
days later, Larry called for an urgent session, having evidently
become involved in treatment.

TREATMENT METHOD: A primary task of the therapist is to
demonstrate effectiveness in response to the patient's behavior
in the initial session. Both interest plus the special skill of
understanding are displayed. These are shown by comments reflecting this understanding and early interpretations of the
issues. Avoiding wild interpretations, but without waiting for
the relationship to develop, the therapist demonstrates his or
her perceptiveness, as well as distinct differences from the others involved with the youngster. By so doing, the therapist
shows confidence in facing the adolescent and the issues so
threatening to him or her. The therapist may describe the basic
conflict as he or she perceives it, for example, or describe the
adolescent's distorted perception of the therapist. The therapist
should be freely able to discuss illegal or embarrassing behavior

in a relaxed manner. The goal is for the impulsive patient to perceive the therapist's perceptiveness and distinctive offers of assistance.

COMMENTARY: This article describes experienced and confident handling of youngsters difficult to engage. With firm early intervention, notable decline in impulsive behavior after involvement in treatment is noted. The newer practitioner must accept that these guidelines, well described, take time to learn to apply effectively. Errors of overinterpretation, pressuring the youngster, or getting drawn into power struggles are common. The authors' interpretations show an empathic response and an ability and willingness to engage in a collaborative look at the problem.

SOURCE: Weinreb, J., and Counts, R. M. "Impulsivity in Adolescents and Its Therapeutic Management." *Archives of General Psychiatry*, 1960, *2*, 548-558.

Additional Readings

Homer, L. E. "Community-Based Resource for Runaway Girls." *Social Casework*, 1973, *54*, 473-479.

There are three popular notions of why adolescents run away: as a cry for help, as an escape from conflict, and as a repudiation of parental values. Twenty girls, thirteen to twenty, repeat runaways referred from juvenile court, received treatment consisting of individual therapy, group counseling, and family therapy. Seven girls were considered to be running from conflicts. Thirteen were viewed as running *to* forbidden experiences: sex, substances of abuse, or a peer group, for example. The "runners from" were more helped by the treatment program. Only four of the thirteen "runners to" were able to respond to the therapist's limit setting. The others were recommended for commitment.

Zastrow, C., and Navarre, R. "Help for Runaways and Their Parents." *Social Casework*, 1975, *56*, 74-78.

Outreach services are offered by this runaway center to youngsters who have run away and do not use clinics or standard service agencies. Emergency shelter and a foster home for up to fourteen days (foster parents were unpaid volunteers) are made available. By law, parents are notified when the child contacts the center. Permission to place the youngster in the foster home is required. Counseling services for the family are available. There are three paid staff and forty volunteer counselors who receive extensive training and supervision. The center is appreciated by the community. After their child's return, parents tend to feel that the problems are unchanged. However, the children report their impression is that the primary problem that led to running is reduced.

◎◎◎◎◎◎◎◎◎◎◎◎◎◎◎◎◎◎◎◎◎◎◎◎◎◎◎◎

Fire Setting

For the protection of the individual and society, an incident of fire setting should be responded to as if it were a call for help (which is often the case). Fire setting has drastically increased in recent years, reflecting the extent of antisocial behavior as a major problem of our time. In adolescents not diagnosed as sociopathic, fire setting has sometimes been related to feelings about family difficulties or occasionally to inappropriate expression of sexual impulses. An extremely thorough assessment of the adolescent is needed as a basis for treatment planning. The question of psychosis and the presence of any feelings of remorse must be determined. In treatment, clear imposition of external controls is usually deemed essential. Parents may be involved in family therapy and also can be helped to set and keep reassuringly firm limits. Residential placement may be necessary for a time, until the evidence suggests that the youngster's impulse control is more secure.

◎◎◎◎◎◎◎◎◎◎◎◎◎◎◎◎◎◎◎◎◎◎◎◎◎◎◎◎

Family and Individual Treatment

AUTHORS: G. A. Awad and S. I. Harrison

PRECIS: A dynamically based model using marital, family, and individual treatment of a female fire setter

INTRODUCTION: Female fire setters are quite rare, and few general conclusions about them are available. Obtaining attention or expressing protest are some suggested underlying meanings of this behavior. In this case report, close attention to familial issues is described. Psychoanalytically based psychiatric treatment was used, with an inpatient and residential phase, in this nonpsychotic early adolescent.

CASE HISTORY: Two prior fires had occurred within a year before Mary, age twelve and a half, confessed to setting fire to curtains in the dining room. Her mother had been talking with a man (possibly her lover) and had just denied Mary's request to go outside. Investigators threatened to remove her to a detention facility unless the family sought help. Mary was hospitalized for evaluation and treatment.

TREATMENT METHOD: Individual, family, and marital therapy were all parts of the treatment. The parents each used individual sessions to air resented facts about the other, which had been believed secret. Such long-standing concerns as her father's doubt of Mary's paternity and her mother's rumored affair, existed in a home atmosphere where these things were not discussed and expression of feelings, including anger, was unacceptable. The therapists saw Mary's fire setting as a burst of anger at her mother, possibly with a sexualized component because her mother's rumored lover was present at the time.

Mary was in residential treatment for a year. In individual therapy, three times weekly, she developed an alliance that enabled her to express her concerns about holding secrets. Frequently, the therapist made comments guessing at her meaning, which she could hear without having to retreat. She would almost never talk directly about fire setting, but it was clear that she did not want to set fires again.

Her problems of extreme dependence upon her mother and extreme sensitivity to her anger and guilt feelings were observed in family sessions. The history of secret keeping made therapeutic steps with the family rather difficult. The parents did come to acknowledge a need to talk and a need for change at home. This allowed Mary some freedom to begin to talk more freely.

TREATMENT RESULTS: The authors suggest that three factors pointed to a favorable prognosis. Mary's ego development was such that she was capable of feeling guilt. Second, although her parents had not paid attention to her problems, they began to show some change, which permitted Mary the chance for freer expression of feelings. Third, Mary was able to respond positively to this more open environment, learning to know when she was angry and express it appropriately.

COMMENTARY: This article gives a clear picture of the dynamics and problems in a single case. The authors advise caution, however, in generalizing conclusions to other cases. They, like others, see fire setting as a behavior with many determinants. In assessing a patient who sets fires, one should consider individual problems, the patient's level of cognitive development, the family style, secondary gain from the behavior, communicative aspects of the symptom, and developmental (pubescent) factors. Although residential treatment may not be necessary in some cases, the drastic initial step of hospitalization communicated to this quite guarded family the seriousness of a long-neglected family problem. Sustained external pressure, such as a court order, may be helpful in maintaining parental support of treatment.

SOURCE: Awad, G. A., and Harrison, S. I. "A Female Fire-Setter: A Case Report." *Journal of Nervous and Mental Disease,* 1976, *163*(6), 432-437.

Fire Fetish Treatment by Multiple
Behavioral Procedures

AUTHOR: S. D. Lande

PRECIS: Orgasmic reconditioning and related techniques to modify arousal reaction to fire-related cognitions

INTRODUCTION: The presenting problems for this late adolescent (age twenty) fire setter were markedly different from the preceding case. Rather than being family related, the major reinforcer for this antisocial act was sexual arousal. The author used several procedures, including a revised version of Marquis's orgasmic reconditioning, that until recently had yielded mixed results. Covert sensitization was also used. The aim was to increase responsiveness to heterosexual stimuli and inhibit sexual arousal to fire-related fantasies.

CASE HISTORY: The patient chose this treatment from among several options after referral by the court for treatment. Twice he had lit a fire in his house, masturbated, and left the house after ejaculation. He still lived with his family. He recalled masturbating to fantasies of houses and cars burning for nearly ten years. At about thirteen he began setting small fires that he put out after masturbating. Fire fantasies still continued, up to five per day. He reported ridicule by peers concerning his clothing and a brace he wore on his leg. Girls rejected him, with one result being that nude photos of women were nonarousing at present. He reported only one (failed) attempt at intercourse, which he had followed up with a fire and masturbation.

TREATMENT METHOD: The therapy plan was to pair sexual arousal, gained from fire stimuli, with female-related material. The aim was to increase association of sexual excitement to heterosexual themes. During pretherapy assessment, the patient was instructed to describe his sexual arousal on a scale from zero (no arousal) to four (most excited) to presented material. In a private room with voice contact, he viewed slides of fires while masturbating. When he was considerably aroused (rating of three or four), he said "switch" and the next slide, a female nude, was presented. The fire slide was shown for a limit of one minute, and the nude for one minute. This sequence was shown five times, then a two-minute rest was given. This constituted an entire sequence. Ten sequences, interrupted by two-minute breaks, were given. He was told to withhold orgasm during this phase. Next he was allowed four minutes to complete orgasm while a nude slide was shown. Assigned "homework" was masturbation while looking at nude pictures. He reported doing this four or five times each week. Four sessions of orgasmic reconditioning were held.

When he reported having sexual fantasies during masturbation, the second phase, covert sensitization, began. He began masturbating to a fire slide for two minutes. While viewing this, a verbal description of an unpleasant reaction to a fire episode (panic, being burned or beaten) was related to him. This cycle was given six times a session for three sessions.

TREATMENT RESULTS: At the end of training, subjective and objective measures of reaction to fire-related material had decreased. Responsiveness to heterosexual erotic material had significantly increased. Gains were maintained at four-month follow-up. He was entered in a group social skills program, not further described in the article. Gains were still present at nine-month follow-up. No fire-setting behavior had recurred.

COMMENTARY: The link between fire setting and sexual arousal, explored in psychoanalytic literature, has been rarely addressed in the more behavioral literature. This revised procedure is a noteworthy addition to the treatment repertoire and may help to increase the use of orgasmic reconditioning, although it has not been widely used. The aversive cognitive element is acceptably mild, in our opinion, with minimal risk. Persons who object to aversive behavior therapies might still find this method acceptable.

SOURCE: Lande, S. D. "A Combination of Orgasmic Reconditioning and Covert Sensitization in the Treatment of a Fire Fetish." *Journal of Behavior Therapy and Experimental Psychiatry,* 1980, *11,* 291-296.

Additional Readings

Eisler, R. M. "Crisis Intervention in the Family of a Firesetter." *Psychotherapy: Theory, Research and Practice,* 1972, *9*(1), 76-79.

A fourteen-year-old, otherwise responsible boy had no explanation for several fires he had set. Disturbed family functioning was explored according to a crisis intervention model, focusing on precipitant factors, role relationships and communication patterns. Six sessions were held, some lasting two or three hours, exploring family fears of expressing negative emotions, helping the father to become more involved and assertive, and other emotionally charged issues. The result was better family functioning, with no recurrence of firesetting at one year followup.

Fine, S., and Louie, D. "Juvenile Firesetters: Do the Agencies Help?" *American Journal of Psychiatry,* 1979, *136,* 433-435.

The authors surveyed the efforts being made to deal with young fire setters in a metropolitan community. The fire marshall, court, and treatment agencies did not systematically coordinate their efforts to deal with the offenders. The two case examples showed multiproblem histories, including lack of parental control, development and school problems, as well as extensive prior agency contact. Their poor adjustment required residential placement. The authors suggest a maximum of six months' trial of community treatment, including intensive parental counseling, with placement as the next step.

Rosenstock, H. A., Holland, A., and Jones, P. H. "Firesetting on an Adolescent Inpatient Unit: An Analysis." *Journal of Clinical Psychiatry,* 1980, *41,* 20-22.

This report describes fire setting on an inpatient unit in three female adolescents with no prior fire setting history. These girls, aged twelve to fifteen, set about five fires in two weeks. Inadequate staff communication or response to the first fire probably led to subsequent incidents. Recent major staff changes and absences were also noted. Recommendations for such situations are clear staff role guidelines for rapid intervention, frequent review of emergencies, and planned activities for relocated patients. Behavior management suggestions include separating the fire setters, ward discussions, and conveying an expectation of a return to safe conditions.

Aggressive Behavior

This section focuses on extremely frequent use of verbal or physical means to attack others. Aggression can follow the loss of self-control or can be a calculated effort to gain an objective after other means have failed. Although aggressive behavior is mentioned in many of the articles included in this book, the ones in this section specifically address aggression as a target for change.

A Social Skills Approach
to Aggression

AUTHORS: J. P. Elder, B. A. Edelstein, and M. M. Narick

PRECIS: Changing aggressive and inappropriate interpersonal
behavior with instructions, modeling, and feedback

INTRODUCTION: These authors demonstrated a generalized
improvement in three target behaviors in youngsters with significant histories of aggression. The procedures required a closely monitored setting, in this case a psychiatric hospital. Methods
were primarily educational, rather than relying on environmental manipulation. Lack of appropriate social skills was viewed as
the prime obstacle to progress.

TREATMENT METHOD: The program was tested on four teenagers in a state hospital adolescent ward. They had been hospitalized for from 2 months to 5 years (mean was 4.9 years). Recently, a ward system with classes, a point-reward system, and a
ward government system had been started. No effect on aggressive behavior had been noted. Two therapists acted as trainers
for the group, which was held in a classroom. Target behaviors,
hypothesized to be related to aggressive behavior, were interrupting others, reactions to others' negative communications,
and asking others to modify their responses.

The group met for forty-five minutes per session, four
times each week. The authors developed eight role-play situations for each one of the target behavior categories. The teenagers contributed typical problem encounters that they faced.
During a pretreatment baseline period (three sessions), each
teenager, with the assistance of a therapist, role played the situations (as many as time would permit). The active treatment
component comprised detailed instructions about each scene,
including possible responses; opportunities to view modeled
examples of successful behavior; and feedback on their performance. Treatment focused on a single target behavior until behavior ratings of their attempts showed major improvement.

Then the next target was addressed. A total of fourteen treatment sessions was required. During this time the rewards and punishment system was not especially changed for these youngsters.

TREATMENT RESULTS: All three target behaviors were improved in the test situation. The most striking results came in nontest situations, showing that the adolescents were successfully applying these new skills. Ward fines for interruptions decreased. Orders for seclusion also declined. Perhaps most notably, three of the teenagers, at three-month follow-up, had been released from the hospital. Six months after that, all three were still in the community. The fourth had reverted to pretreatment behavior.

COMMENTARY: Several factors probably contributed to the success of this program. The new ward system, based on the Achievement Place model, seems to have brought improved consequences to behavior to the ward. It might have introduced a noticeable external pressure on adolescents, necessary for effective ward interventions, such as this aggression-reducing program. The extent of the generalization was impressive, as were the gains, considering the chronicity of their illnesses.

SOURCE: Elder, J. P., Edelstein, B. A., and Narick, M. M. "Modifying Aggressive Behavior with Social Skills Training." *Behavior Modification,* 1979, *3*(2), 161-178.

Reducing Assaultive Behavior by a Self-Control Procedure

AUTHOR: S. I. Pfeiffer

PRECIS: Physical and verbal aggression eliminated by behavior rehearsal and self-control techniques

INTRODUCTION: Self-control improvement techniques have been applied to a wide variety of behaviors, including obsessive-compulsive acts and weight loss. This work with a student complaining of uncontrollable aggressive and verbal acts was done in a high school setting.

CASE HISTORY: A nineteen-year-old senior was referred by a guidance counselor to the school psychologist. He had been repeatedly observed to physically attack his girlfriend, also a student at the school. In the first contact with the therapist, the goal was defined as planning a way to improve his "temper." The suggestion was made that self-control procedures be tried, and the model was described. The student agreed to the proposal. The next step was a behavior analysis, in which information was gathered about the aggression. This included a clear description of the undesirable behaviors, frequency, intensity, duration, place of occurrence, presence of other people, and consequences of the act. It should be noted that in this case the girlfriend's and family's cooperation was not requested.

TREATMENT METHOD: The client's first task was to make a frequency count, that is, how many times each day he performed each targeted problem behavior. Instructions were given on how to record this. Also, an anecdotal summary of each incident was requested for the first week. A review of these showed the two most troublesome behaviors to be hitting his girlfriend and verbal aggression toward his girlfriend and parents. Hitting, the target behavior showing least self-control, was the first behavior considered.

The procedure was the same for both behaviors, however. It consisted of three parts:

1. Instruction about the appropriate learning theory model of behavior. Initially, readings were assigned, but the student failed to complete them, giving the burden of schoolwork as his reason. The plan was changed; the therapist devoted a part of each of the eight sessions to presenting applications of learning theory to problem behaviors.

2. A graded series, that is, gradually increasing in intensity, of aggression-provoking situations was developed for role-playing purposes.

3. The student was trained in self-control techniques. *Response inhibition* was defined as refraining from overt action for approximately one minute at the onset of an event that usually would lead to aggression. *Cognitive intervention* consisted of subvocal statements of guilt feelings that could be expected if he acted on his aggressive feelings. *Covert reinforcement* was self-administered praise for refraining from aggressive acts.

The procedure was first implemented on physical events only, for four sessions, with no discussions of verbal aggression. After that, the application to verbal aggression was begun.

TREATMENT RESULTS: Results from self-report showed complete elimination of physical aggression after the start of the procedure. After the verbal aggression part of the program began, incidence of this behavior dropped 80 percent. The data were confirmed by the girlfriend, family, and teacher. Six-month and one-year follow-up showed that behavior remained at the same posttreatment level.

COMMENTARY: This report is a good example of the adaptability of self-control procedures to a variety of behaviors and settings. Several features of self-control procedures are illustrated here, including flexibility in choice of procedures. Some possible additional methods used in development of self-control with problem behaviors include thought stopping, covert modeling, and imagery techniques.

The therapist's rapid response to the client's unwillingness to read assigned material is especially noteworthy. From this, the therapist clearly did *not* conclude that this early response indicated decreased motivation or resistance to treatment. Instead, the approach was changed to better suit the client's circumstances. The same data, on behavioral principles, was learned in a different manner. An interesting feature of this program is that outside support for the treatment program was not required from important people in the client's life. However, the client showed good motivation for change, completing most of the work with little reported difficulty.

SOURCE: Pfeiffer, S. I. "A School Psychologist's Use of Short-Term Behavior Therapy in a High School Setting." *Psychology*, 1977, *14*, 40-44.

Additional Reading

Goldstein, A. P., Sherman, M., Gershaw, N. J., Sprafkin, R. P., and Glick, B. "Training Aggressive Adolescents in Prosocial Behavior." *Journal of Youth and Adolescence*, 1978, *7*, 73-92.

The authors posit a behavior deficiency model of adolescent aggression. Certain socially needed behaviors are not even weakly present; so the first step is skill training. Structured Learning Therapy (SLT) uses modeling, role playing, social reinforcement, and transfer of learning to other situations. Practice and overlearning are considered essential. This work is part of an extensive project to develop skill training in a wide range of behaviors (see A. P. Goldstein, R. P. Sprafkin, and N. J. Gershaw, *Skill Training for Community Living: Applying Structured Learning Therapy*, New York: Pergamon Press, 1976).

@@

Acting Out

From its origin in psychoanalytic usage, this term has come to be employed in describing a variety of impulsive acts, sometimes antisocial, sometimes self-destructive. This section focuses on the acting-out process present in adolescents described in many sections of this book.

At first, acting out applied to persons with strong ego controls who at stressful points in therapy expressed or repeated a past event in action rather than admit it to consciousness. Current use of the term includes repetitive acts occurring outside of treatment in more poorly controlled persons. Attempts at relief by action of inner distress usually provide temporary respite at best. These acts are often viewed as attempts to change a part of reality that is perceived as the cause of the trouble while denying personal responsibility. Frequently the result of this is additional difficulty, because the individual's impulsiveness does not permit consideration of all the consequences of the action.

@@

A Psychoanalytic Approach to the
Acting-Out Adolescent

AUTHOR: J. F. Masterson

PRECIS: Management and treatment of acting out in a border-line teen

INTRODUCTION: The author describes the psychodynamic mechanisms in the acting-out process and the resulting treatment problems. The denial of problems and projection of blame and responsibility for one's problems are the basis for the teenager's view of the problems and the unhelpful world. As a result, the attempts to act out, which provide brief relief, seem inappropriate only to the observer. What the adolescent cannot perceive is that the acting out is an attempted solution to a perceptual recreation of a long-standing, infancy-based, distressing situation.

CASE HISTORY: Sixteen-year-old Frank, a high school junior, had been acting out against his mother for about a year, fighting with her, taking a variety of drugs, being truant and unproductive in school. He was to be seen three times weekly, with his parents seeing a social worker once weekly. Frank was to pay $15 weekly toward the treatment costs.

TREATMENT METHOD: In the therapy of these patients, therapist and patient hold incompatible conceptions of both problem and solutions, making communication almost impossible. The patient sees therapy as an adversary process. Manipulation and deception are means to avoid frustration, which is the most intolerable possibility. Manipulation and deception are used to control the therapy. Denial of an act's consequences, inability to see a relation between feelings and behavior or between past, present, and future are common.

It is sometimes helpful to view the patient's perceptions and the acting out as an art form. This acknowledges the primitive level of cognition and the prominence of impulse. It may also increase a therapist's interest level in the patient's dynamics while reducing anger at the oppositional and impulsive turns taken in treatment.

Masterson's guidelines on management were developed with borderline acting-out adolescents but may apply to other diagnostic groups. They are based on his conclusions about the early chronic problems that are the basis of borderline dynamics. During the period of eighteen to thirty-six months, a loss of relationship with the mother causes proneness to depression and fixation on the loss of this relationship. In adolescence, the fixation remains the primary problem, with acting out as the defense against the depressive experience of abandonment. To the patient, forming a therapeutic relationship increases chances of being abandoned again; therefore this must be resisted. The therapist's work toward forming this alliance includes confronting these adversary defensive actions. If the adolescent is in a closed setting, limit setting can be used with good effects.

In beginning treatment, time is a problem in several ways. The adolescent is usually at some further risk of acting out. If the therapist does not quickly respond to the patient's early defensive maneuvers, increased resistance or abandonment of therapy may result. Accordingly, limit setting must be done at the earliest juncture, before a positive transferential relationship is formed. This works surprisingly well, helping to strengthen the adolescent's weak understanding of how dangerous the acting out really is. Another benefit is that the adolescent, equating lack of parental discipline with loss of interest, interprets the therapist's behavior as genuine interest.

By the fifth session, Frank was gleefully castigating his mother when the therapist began limit setting by disturbing his happy mood. Suggesting Frank was trying to avoid depressive feelings he couldn't comprehend, the therapist noted that it was too simple to explain all Frank's problems as due to his mother. Frank confirmed this by saying his poor schoolwork was to get back at his mother. The therapist's response was to point out the sad aspect of such self-destructive behavior. When Frank doubted he could control his anger unless he could see the therapist immediately, the response was to point out the long-term nature of the problems and the unreality of asking for quick fixes.

Although the therapist was verbally active, he did not ask many questions, which Frank resented because he had to do more work. He didn't want to pay his share and was reminded that the payment represented a measure of independence and self-respect, which he wouldn't get by buying drugs instead. At home, in an outburst against his previous pattern of overcompliance, he wrote obscenities on his walls and attempted to provoke termination of treatment.

The therapist spoke at length about the empty feelings when the alternatives in life were drugs or boredom. His recent loss of interests and hobbies was reviewed, and the hope of pleasures that required time and effort was extended. Soon Frank responded by expressing his depression and a sense that he was missing something. He wanted help and said the therapist wasn't giving any. Again the demand for instant help or "no dice" was noted, and ways of being effectively, less destructively independent were raised.

TREATMENT RESULTS: Although Frank continued to bring back the same themes, his testing of the therapist declined as he was able to verbalize the depressive aspects of his relations with his parents. The effective limit setting was apparently the basis for the development of his confidence in the therapist.

COMMENTARY: The difficulty of working with acting-out youngsters and the activity required of the therapist is well described in this article. By demanding that the therapist conduct the treatment in a certain way (for example, questions), the youngster attempts to replicate the hated chronic fantasy and then to use his accustomed defenses. However, the therapist's assertive responses and demonstration of the help to be gained from verbal expression of conflicts are key factors in success.

SOURCE: Masterson, J. F. "The Acting-Out Adolescent: A Point of View." *American Journal of Psychotherapy*, 1974, *28*, 343-351.

A Multiple Approach Stressing Individual Therapy and External Controls

AUTHOR: J. Chwast

PRECIS: Elements of successful therapy with severely acting-out teenagers

INTRODUCTION: Acting out, or externalized expression of psychological conflict in an inappropriate fashion, is a frequent aspect of adolescent behavior, especially in our times. A permissive society produces situations requiring greater self-control. This can be especially difficult for, among others, emotionally disturbed and environmentally deprived adolescents. Living in socially or financially stressed families, they see a more affluent surrounding while having very few resources themselves. Some teenagers respond to this disparity with antisocial action. Impulsive, aggressive, hostile behavior may reduce anxiety, forestall the need of verbal interchange, and avoid feelings of envy, guilt, depression, or hopelessness. This pattern may in turn result in arrest and court-ordered treatment.

TREATMENT METHOD: The primary goal of involuntary or semivoluntary treatment is development of useful self-generated behavior control. Chwast's method for achieving this requires, first, an effective external pressure, such as court threat, to make sure the therapeutic process can be begun. Second, a clear link is needed between the therapist and the external authority (probation officer, for example) to promote accountability and rapid response to the patient's acts.

Two issues that must be handled at the early stage of treatment are clarifying the nature of the therapeutic contract and setting realistic early goals to respond to aspects of the situation (such as family difficulties) that are still in a crisis situation. Chwast feels that clinics and agencies can be set up to handle these cases well. Paraprofessionals employed by the clinic can also be useful. They can help the acting-out youngster arrange aspects of his or her outside life, including finding a job.

Several general guidelines for the therapist are offered. Three ingredients are vital to the therapy process. The first is control. The therapist should remember and not be reluctant to use the authority over the teenager's future. One can increase or decrease pressure, as needed, for the teenager to keep up work at agreed upon activities. This includes attendance at therapy sessions. Having to use this power is one of several ways that the therapist's countertransference feelings are aroused. The teenager's threatening, telling half-truths or out-right lies, and accusing the therapist of telling outsiders private material all contribute to evoking strong reactions in the therapist. Demonstrating that one is aware of these behaviors and their probable motives helps to strengthen the therapist's control of the situation.

The second ingredient is support. This can consist of assistance in getting a job or a school program settled or in negotiating a conditional arrangement with an agency or authority and active efforts early in treatment to help assure the survival and protection of the young client.

The third ingredient is uncovering. This self-discovery process is known to be especially anxiety producing in the adolescent. Too often the patient settles for a glib statement, which proves to be superficial, as evidence of insight. The therapist is advised to offer small but consistently aggressive statements for the patient to work with. This not only shows the therapist's skill to the patient but also introduces a more valid understanding of the patient's world.

Chwast warns us not to lose sight of the unstable nature of the acting-out patient. This person has typically found social agencies unresponsive in the past and has fared poorly. Patients' life situations often call for activity or advocacy by the professional to secure improved agreements with the service or legal agencies with which they cope. Paraprofessionals or other agency personnel can help with this.

COMMENTARY: In this and his other articles (see Additional Readings in the Delinquency section), Chwast helps us to design and implement an affective therapy model for vigorously resistive adolescents. They require enough control to keep them safe and able to remain in the treatment situation, instead of being removed for placement. He illustrates the needed link between social therapy, which provides the needed external authority, and concomitant technical psychotherapy issues. Many professionals are hesitant about working with such clients, as sessions may prove quite stressful. This is an example of productive developments with populations in great need of help.

SOURCE: Chwast, J. "Psychotherapy of Disadvantaged Acting-Out Adolescents." *American Journal of Psychotherapy,* 1977, *31,* 216-226.

Use of Rational Behavior Therapy

AUTHOR: M. C. Maultsby, Jr.

PRECIS: Teaching the relation between irrational thinking and its consequences for acting out

INTRODUCTION: Some diagnostic criteria and a rational behavior therapy sequence for acting-out behavior are offered in this article. Maultsby suggests the acting-out pattern exists in the following situations for nonpsychotic, nonretarded teens:

1. If guilt acts as a stimulus to further disruptions, rather than leading to apology or compromise (as in the normal adolescent)
2. Where emotional conflict of some duration is clearly present (rather than absent, as in the case of the antisocial personality)

CASE HISTORY: Richard had recently been depressed, and it was with no warning that he was arrested, along with three others, for stripping cars. Therapy was mandated as a condition of probation.

TREATMENT METHOD: The author defines the first major task in treatment as identifying the emotional conflict and providing a resolution. The tenets of rational behavior therapy, described in many articles, are employed here to achieve a working description of the acting-out behavior as a logical result of an emotional turmoil. This turmoil is based on faulty or inadequate percepts or thinking habits. Improvements in these maladaptive thinking patterns should reduce or eliminate outbursts.

Part of Richard's treatment was to learn the features of rational thinking. The necessary criteria of (1) relationship to objective facts, (2) a self-protective aspect, (3) relation to the person's objective self-interest, and its helping to minimize (4) intrapsychic or (5) interpersonal conflict were taught. He learned that what he called facts had included many subjective distortions, with his emotions having changed his statements to himself and others. A major goal was to achieve mastery of irrational thinking. One way of doing this was to learn the method of rational self-analysis (RSA). This was then used to examine his attachment to the group, which he had rejoined despite his disapproval of their stealing.

First, he wrote down the event as objectively as possible: *He left the gang, because they stole, but they jeered at him, which hurt his feelings; so he asked to come back.*

Second, he wrote his thoughts about it: *He couldn't tolerate stealing. It was imperative to leave.*

Third, he wrote his subsequent feelings about it: *He felt like a "dirty rat" for leaving his friends.*

Fourth, he reviewed the first two steps with the therapist's assistance, clarifying which aspects were not in fact rational. Regarding the first, he came to see that being called names had not hurt him. To waste time believing that the names applied to him was irrational. Regarding the second, it was clarified that he *had* tolerated stealing, and his behavior indicated that he *didn't* have to leave. His actions were out of line with his own professed values.

Fifth, he tried to anticipate what would be the emotional results of his behavior if it were more along the lines suggested by the fourth step. *It would be unimportant what thieves felt*

about him. He could have more self-esteem. This allowed for
the third step to be reviewed and revised.

TREATMENT RESULTS: At first Richard thought RSA was
little more than word play. As he came to see how his irrational
assumptions had led to inappropriate conclusions, feelings, and
actions, he became enthusiastically involved. He did two or
more RSA sequences weekly through three months of individual rational behavior therapy. Following a switch to three
months of group rational behavior therapy, treatment was considered completed. Follow-up information showed that Richard
successfully completed probation, then high school. At last
word he was doing well in college.

COMMENTARY: As used here, RSA helps to expose and explore the gap between the patient's statements of belief and the
contrasting evidence from observed behavior. This method gives
a direct experience of the difference between facts and the subjective implications attributed to them. This distinction is easily
blurred and causes much pain in many normal teenagers. The
fusion of fact and irrational implication is especially seen in acting out. This method helps to counter the reinforcing properties
of acting out as described by Maultsby—temporary alleviation
of the pressure of conflict, without the pain of change. It offered this acting-out adolescent a coherent, alternative view of
the choices and judgments that he made without being aware of
it. The rational self-analysis system, based on the work of Al-
bert Ellis, should be thoroughly studied before being introduced.

SOURCE: Maultsby, M. C., Jr. "Rational Behavior Therapy for
   Acting-Out Adolescents." *Social Casework*, 1975, *56*, 35-43.

Exploring Family Dynamics
in Acting Out

AUTHORS: G. Schneiderman and H. Evans

PRECIS: Reducing the behavior impulses by exploring family feelings of emotional deprivation

INTRODUCTION: The authors treated with family therapy a teen found stealing. Special attention was paid to the stealing as a symptom expressive of a wish. Schneiderman and Evans note a tendency in families of acting-out adolescents to terminate treatment at a very early point. They present an explanation for this and a treatment alternative. The problem, as they viewed it, lies with interpretations stressing the aggressive nature of the act. In such situations, their recommendation is to explore feelings of need and deprivation before making aggressiveness-related interpretations. This can lead to learning what people in the family want from each other. Later, aggressive aspects can be explored.

CASE HISTORY: Paul, fifteen, the oldest of four children, had stolen on several occasions. His school performance was also poor. Paul's father was observed to be complaining but rather weak. His mother complained about Paul's and her husband's past failures. The parents' own histories showed lack of a close, affectionate relationship with the same-sex parent. The therapists hypothesized that all three, Paul and parents, still felt unable to accept the lack of such a relationship. Paul's stealing was a symbolic attempt to make up for this felt loss.

TREATMENT METHOD: Early family sessions were accusatory. The father endorsed the mother's critical remarks about Paul. He criticized her punishments as inappropriate, whereupon she attacked him and a marital squabble ensued. Early therapist interventions addressed Paul's anger at being denied a warmer relationship with his parents. The family apparently accepted this as correct, but shortly afterwards attempted to stop treatment.

The accusations and the interpretations, the therapists realized, had stimulated feelings of guilt and responsibility in the parents. Unable to manage these feelings, they attempted to leave. The therapists changed their remarks to focus on the equally accessible feelings of loss and affectional needs. Paul was presenting as wanting affection, rather than accusing his parents of not offering it. All family members were able to respond to this and treatment continued. Members were encouraged to explore their wishes for communication, attention, and love within the family. Problems in receiving and giving affection were raised and solutions were offered.

TREATMENT RESULTS: With increased confidence in their ability to relate successfully, they began to express anger. At this point, Paul's cessation of stealing and better schoolwork were reported. The parents continued to work toward the father's more active involvement and a more receptive toleration of this by his wife.

COMMENTARY: The authors' experience illustrates the sequential nature of rebuilding family relations. This family needed an alternative to stealing and recrimination. Therapists need to deflect this negative behavior and provide a better therapeutic focus. Focus on need provides a topic to which all can relate, increasing commitment to therapy. An important goal of this approach is the recognition of the family members' own ability to change their relations and solve problems. The premature expression of anger in the therapeutic milieu can be, and in this case almost was, destructive of treatment.

SOURCE: Schneiderman, G., and Evans, H. "An Approach to Families of Acting-Out Adolescents—A Case Study." *Adolescence,* 1975, *10*(40), 495-498.

Additional Readings

Elitzur, B. "Self-Relaxation Program for Acting-Out Adolescents." *Adolescence,* 1976, *11*(44), 569-572.

This method was developed for twelve- to sixteen-year-olds who committed probation violations or other acts requiring temporary removal from their families. Placed in short-term shelters, they often showed major emotional reactions to this drastic step. Relaxation as a group activity was offered on a voluntary basis to ease adjustment to the situation. The time of day selected for teaching was about 3 P.M., on the basis of staff opinion that youngsters were most irritable at this time. Group instruction was given with the goal of teaching voluntary self-relaxation to encourage independent use of the procedure. An auxiliary instruction tape was available for use when the need to relax was felt. Staff felt that youngsters who attended the relaxation program had fewer adjustment problems, although supportive data were not available. The youngsters reported feeling better and had varied positive descriptions of their feelings during relaxation.

Johnson, A. M., and Szurek, S. A. "The Genesis of Antisocial Acting Out in Children and Adults." *Psychoanalytic Quarterly,* 1952, *21*, 323-343.

Certain youngsters show a limited acting-out pattern within a generally well-adjusted pattern. These narrow problems reflect "superego lacunae" in people who have a largely effective superego. In this classic paper, the acting-out behavior is interpreted as assisting parents to obtain vicarious gratification of their own poorly handled impulses. Feelings of guilt in the youngster seem to be blocked by a sense of having permission by the parents to act out. Understanding of the dynamics usually requires exchange of information by therapists of both parent and child. Treatment involves a positive, often dependent relationship to the therapist, assistance in tolerating guilt, and improved ability to perceive one's actions realistically.

Lulow, W. V. "Therapeutic Technique: Treatment of a Borderline Adolescent Girl." *American Journal of Psychotherapy,* 1977, *31*, 366-375.

The author treated a severely disturbed, acting-out thirteen-year-old girl. She used drugs, was self-destructive, and was described diagnostically as borderline. The therapist saw her three times weekly with weekly parental counseling by another therapist. A major treatment tool was confrontation. When Jane insisted on fewer sessions, the therapist suggested her ability to judge this was not as good as the doctor's. Her treatment exemplified the dangers of being a "nice guy" therapist, for whom acting-out patients often feel contempt. The therapist needed to demonstrate his capacity to handle the patient's negativity and also respond effectively to her narcissistic needs. Therapy required effective responses to testing, willingness to make suggestions without expecting a response, inquiring into self-destructive episodes, showing concern, and calling for her to be more intelligently concerned about herself. The parents' therapist encouraged more responsible discipline at home. The two therapists shared a goal of increased psychological separation of mother and daughter.

Minuchin, S., Auerswald, E., King, C. H., and Rabinowitz, C. "The Study and Treatment of Families that Produce Multiple Acting-Out Boys." *American Journal of Orthopsychiatry,* 1964, *34,* 125-133.

In working with disturbed youngsters in residential treatment and their families, Minuchin et al. stress that the chief complaints regarding the boys must be considered *family problems.* This must be made clear at the first session. Helpful techniques have included holding one or two sessions in the home and energetic assistance in some life problems, such as getting babysitters, shoes, or assisting a move. In family sessions lasting up to two hours, two therapists first see the entire family together with the child's therapist. In the second phase, parents are seen separately, as is the sibling group. After discussion, all parties reassemble. The therapists require a postgroup review. Families are seen for about twenty-five to thirty sessions.

Treatment of Predelinquents and Early Delinquents

Several criteria are commonly employed in classifying youngsters under these headings. First offenders or frequent minor offenders are often referred to in this way. A younger adolescent is more likely to receive this description than a more serious label. Lastly, these teens have not been formally adjudicated.

Youngsters in this category are considered to be at risk, in danger of involvement in more serious crime, and requiring help. Two important themes are to be noted in the following articles. One is the strategy of rapid, active intervention, with utilization of therapeutic and community service resources. The second is the theme of therapy or activities programs as having a preventive effect.

Crisis Intervention

AUTHOR: J. G. Stratton

PRECIS: Reducing recidivism in minor offenders by a family counseling approach at the time of arrest

INTRODUCTION: According to Stratton, effective intervention in crises should leave the client better able to cope when the immediate problem has been resolved. Counseling families in crises has been increasingly employed in preventive fashion in the community, using specially trained police, for example. The author is a psychologist in a county sheriff's office in a large metropolitan area. For families whose teenage child has already been arrested, the issue is whether counseling at this disturbing time would be effective. The goal of this study was to resolve contributory family factors and reduce recidivism.

TREATMENT METHOD: The methods used here were tested on youngsters in two categories: those whose charges would be misdemeanors in an adult and youngsters with predelinquent type offenses, including truancy, runaway behavior, and similar out of control acts. The intervention counselors (one psychologist and another worker trained and supervised by him) saw thirty families. Thirty other families, handled in the standard fashion, constituted a comparison group. The principles and methods were as follows:

1. Swift response (first session preferably within one to two hours of arrest).
2. Vigorous expression by the counselor of his or her views.
3. Primary emphasis on the current problems of all family members. (This required a problem-solving procedure utilizing exploration of the current major crisis, venting of feelings related to the arrest, review of prior attempted solutions with emphasis on why they were unsuccessful, and pressing for plans for the youngster and family to try new approaches.)

4. A minimum of one follow-up meeting (average of 2.5 sessions).

5. Option to contact the counselor in case of later problems.

The families of the arrested minors often had severe handicaps or were in a state of considerable disorganization. For example, both parents of one fourteen-year-old runaway were blind, and he felt an overwhelming burden of seeing for three people. Their anxiety about the world was a pressure with which he could not cope. The thrust of counseling for him was learning alternative possibilities to running away from the extremely frustrating life situation. The beginnings of better dialogue with his parents were also noted at this session.

In another example, a sixteen-year-old boy was evicted by both his parents and shunted between two other relatives. Here the counselor's focus was on how little help the boy could expect from his estranged family and on how to make some difficult decisions in spite of this.

TREATMENT RESULTS: Evaluation of the program showed that the community valued the police station counseling service. Stratton's own data supported the program to a moderate extent. In contrast to the comparison group, the youngsters in the counseling program committed fewer subsequent crimes. Less probation department involvement was needed, and all services for the counseled families averaged less than half that required for the comparison group families. It was noted that some additional counselor time was required to respond to those who missed appointments by going to the home. This was especially important in the cases of families without telephones or transportation.

A common point noted by the counselor was the frequently expressed wish of families that the counselors or police would take over the entire problem. Active intervention by the counselor was needed to change this viewpoint and get the family to work together.

COMMENTARY: This is clearly an innovative program of therapeutic value. A notable feature is Stratton's goal: that crisis counseling rather than simply a "quick fix" should significantly reduce future troublesome behavior. Crisis or preventive intervention, besides being a bona fide therapy service, is usually cost-effective. As Stratton showed, it reduces future use of government agency time for repeat offenders. Further, paraprofessionals can also be trained and supervised by professional therapists in this work. This is an important way of providing treatment service to young offenders and their families.

SOURCE: Stratton, J. G. "Effects of Crisis Intervention Counseling on Predelinquent and Misdemeanor Juvenile Offenders." *Juvenile Justice*, 1975, *3*, 7-18.

Family Contracting and Self-Reinforcement in a Case of Stealing

AUTHOR: J. S. Stumphauzer

PRECIS: Changing individual and family patterns in the case of an early adolescent girl

INTRODUCTION: Stealing by adolescents is a common problem that has received few claims of successful treatment. The act results in immediate positive reinforcement—acquisition of a desired object. Aversive factors that might reduce stealing, such as punishments or legal procedures, are slow, inconsistently delivered, and have a weak effect. The case reported here uses behavior analysis to diagnose the situation, with self-control training and family contingency contracting to control the behavior.

CASE HISTORY: This twelve-year-old black girl was referred by parochial officials after a five-year history of stealing. She took various items almost every day. Both school officials and parents collaborated to keep her behavior away from public notice, with the result that she was watched closely, isolated, and rarely allowed out alone. There were no other antisocial behaviors. Behavior analysis led to several conclusions. First, she received much attention, not all negative, after discovery. Her mother smiled while describing the problem. Parental response was inconsistent, consisting of restriction or prayer. They suggested her problem was due to a "sickness." Because sweets were often taken, her father believed she was diabetic. The therapist concluded that stealing was maintained strongly by attention and reward. Further, little positive response to more socially acceptable behavior was available to her.

The therapist thought she took pleasure in pleasing others and showed some motivation to stop stealing. Further, she was intelligent and liked school. However, like her parents, she felt she couldn't control her stealing.

TREATMENT METHOD: Treatment began with three sessions of behavior analysis. The mother and the teacher completed daily behavior rating forms on frequency of stealing. At the same time, diabetes was ruled out by medical examination, leading the parents to respond more to the current approach. The girl herself was taught self-control according to the program developed by Kanfer and Karoly (F. H. Kanfer and P. Karoly, "Self-control: a Behavioristic Excursion into the Lion's Den," *Behavior Therapy*, 1972, *3*, 398-416). Elements of this program were self-monitoring, self-evaluation, and self-reinforcement. First, beginning with the fourth session, she measured her own stealing on a behavior chart. Self-evaluation occurred when she summarized her behavior, including whether she was thinking of stealing. She role played alternative behaviors that would help her focus away from stealing. Self-reinforcement included many positive statements she could make when she refrained from stealing. She could make self-reinforcing comments immediately and more general statements about her improvement at other times, including periods of indecision.

TREATMENT RESULTS: The family and school personnel,

after consultation, were able to shift their attention to her non-stealing behaviors, especially her behaviors that were incompatible with stealing. Further, a family contract gave her twenty cents for each day of no stealing, plus special weekend activities and meals for each theft-free week. The program also treated her social isolation. When she had achieved partial control, trips to the store to buy an item were begun. At first she took her little sister, but she later made many other trips alone. The family was then able to encourage and praise outside independent activity. Follow-up at six, twelve, and eighteen months showed no stealing. Her mother had confidence in her and felt she did not need careful watching anymore. She had continued to develop outside interests.

COMMENTARY: Because this stealing pattern is not usual, the author suggests caution in applying this method without prior behavior analysis. The girl, the family, and the school all expressed some concern. This program can be offered if the youngster is open to offers of help in obtaining mastery over impulses. It is not clear if, with school and family cooperation, this program would be applicable for a less motivated, antisocial youngster.

SOURCE: Stumphauzer, J. S. "Elimination of Stealing by Self-Reinforcement of Alternative Behavior and Family Contracting." *Journal of Behavior Therapy and Experimental Psychiatry*, 1976, 7, 265-268.

Behavioral Goal-Oriented Modification of Family Interaction Style

AUTHORS: J. F. Alexander and B. V. Parsons

PRECIS: Reduced recidivism through family communication training

INTRODUCTION: The authors' starting point was a research finding demonstrating that families of delinquents had different conversation patterns. There was less talk, with strikingly unequal participation in these families. The therapists' goal was to normalize this pattern in referred families, using a brief treatment model. An extensive evaluation program examined the treatment program's effects.

TREATMENT METHOD: The families in the project were referred from the county juvenile court. The adolescents' behaviors included truancy, running away, shoplifting, and possessing soft drugs or alcohol. The adolescents ranged in age from thirteen to sixteen. The therapists, graduate students in clinical psychology, received extensive training and supervision.

Goals set for families were better communication, including more evenly distributed contributions and better give and take, as well as improved behavior management skills. The families were presented with the idea that their unsatisfactory interchanges made their adolescent's offending behavior more likely. The suggestion was offered that learning to arrange agreements within the family could effectively remove a major contributor to the problem situations. They encouraged attempts to negotiate agreements. Because the major offenses were too difficult to begin with, less sensitive issues were selected as targets for first negotiation.

Using modeling and verbal reinforcements, therapists taught discussion skills, including clear statement of issues as well as one's feelings, presenting demands, offering alternatives, and fixing costs for privileges and rewards for assuming responsibilities. The training sessions were held over a five- or six-week period.

In addition, communication conventions were defined for the family. A "rule" was aimed at controlling and limiting. It was to be clearly distinguished from a "request." Requests were not supposed to carry threat of punishment if refused.

The therapists defined several other communication patterns. They taught methods of interrupting to clarify an issue, to add information, to share one's feelings or opinions on a topic, and to give feedback to other family members. The therapists praised effective interruptions.

TREATMENT RESULTS: Results showed that family interactions were significantly changed. Interaction was more evenly distributed among family members on posttest evaluation. There was less silence, suggesting greater family investment in interaction. Interruptions had increased during this time. Court records showed that subsequent referrals of these youngsters for behavior or criminal offenses were significantly less than for groups treated by a comparison treatment and a nontreatment control group.

COMMENTARY: Court-related intervention programs utilize the crisis situation caused by the adolescent's arrest to achieve a more effective intervention. The present program is distinguished by its skill development emphasis, rather than focusing on alleviation of acute precipitants. Although recidivism was still present (at a 25 percent rate), this program was probably cost-effective in terms of less subsequent involvement with the majority of youngsters. Projects such as this should be considered as both treatment and community delinquency prevention programs, as they may serve to reduce the likelihood of further, more major acts.

SOURCE: Alexander, J. F., and Parsons, B. V. "Short-Term Behavioral Intervention with Delinquent Families: Impact on Family Process and Recidivism." *Journal of Abnormal Psychology*, 1973, *81*, 219-223.

Mandated Group Therapy for Minor Offenders and Their Parents

AUTHORS: E. H. Steininger and L. Leppel

PRECIS: Selection of youthful offenders in a probation-related project

INTRODUCTION: Juvenile offenders often fail to follow through on court referrals for treatment. If an initial appointment is kept, early disinterest, noncooperation, and resentment are common. When things quiet down, people stop coming. The method described here maintains pressure on families to stay in treatment. There is also a built-in follow-up procedure. The program goals are reduced recidivism and improved community adjustment.

TREATMENT METHOD: The juvenile probation officers were advised to refer juvenile offenders and their families to the program and to insist on attendance if accepted. The program was refined over a two-year period. Youths who had been charged with only one or two offenses were selected. Originally, hard core multiple offenders had been referred but proved not to be helped much by the program. The best results seemed to accrue to those under sixteen.

In the final form of the group, the youngster and at least one parent had to be screened for the group. All were interviewed individually, the parents filled out a family background questionnaire, and the children were briefly tested. Psychotic and mentally retarded adolescents were not accepted.

Boys were placed in groups of five or six. Parents were seen in separate groups of similar size. An attempt to get both parents to work together in the group was not successful. Enough males were present, however, to make possible discussion of father and mother roles. The client families were seen for up to a maximum of thirty-four sessions.

Both boys' and parents' groups showed capability of cohesive work and interest in others' problems. Parents used many sessions to ventilate anger toward their children, school and police authorities, and having to come to sessions. The white children were able to discuss their families, but the black youngsters did so rarely. Later groups formed were less successful in keeping black families in the program, for unclear reasons. In both groups, episodes of open expression of feelings and problems were usually followed by absence or nonparticipation the following week.

TREATMENT RESULTS: The second group of boys, the minor offenders, showed the most optimistic results. Only two of the eight boys who completed the program were brought back to court within the following year.

COMMENTARY: Use of treatment programs with a "coercive" attendance component is still being debated at this point in the development of therapies for delinquent adolescents. Two facts should be noted. In this program no penalties were imposed if a family dropped out. Further, the results of this and similar programs reported elsewhere in this chapter suggest that common pessimistic predictions about outcome are not founded. Unmotivated offenders need some extra help to begin working in their rehabilitation, and pressure to attend is one way to supply this.

SOURCE: Steininger, E. H., and Leppel, L. "Group Therapy for Reluctant Juvenile Probationers and Their Parents." *Adolescence*, 1970, 5(17), 67-78.

Psychodrama Treatment with Delinquents

AUTHORS: P. Carpenter and S. Sandberg

PRECIS: Increasing communication skills and expression of blocked feelings in a delinquent group

INTRODUCTION: The authors list common social and emotional deficits found in delinquents. Poor communication skills, minimal display of empathy, guarded attitudes, and inability to employ fantasy were considered target behaviors for treatment. Although not the cause of their being arrested, these lacks were considered hindrances to the development of greater prosocial behavior. Employment of fantasy was considered an important potential alternative to direct action without forethought, a common response in delinquents.

TREATMENT METHOD: The county juvenile court maintained a clinic for children referred for school, community, and domestic problems ranging from fighting to theft and sex offenses. Sixteen delinquents, aged fifteen to sixteen, were formed into a thirty-session psychodrama group. Many techniques derived by J. L. Moreno, founder of psychodrama, were used, but only a few of the notably effective were described in this article. Atmosphere was important. Use of dim light seemed to have a relaxing effect on members, who related more easily in the dim atmosphere.

Through experimentation, it became clear that structure had to be imposed on the session. A warm-up, with directed exercises, and exploration of a theme selected by the leader from the responses in the warm-up, was the usual format. Allowing the members to raise issues or choose roles was unproductive. Warm-up exercises might consist of music, poetry, or the notably effective "magic shop," in which members came to the "store" to order anything they wanted. Some ordered friends or love, setting up a scene that could be psychodramatically elaborated. Wishes could be expressed and explored, with no action necessary. This gave these youngsters a rare experience of expressing a need without acting impulsively on these wishes.

Poetry readings were eagerly responded to, and youngsters began to bring in their own selections. A poignant example, written by a girl shortly before her suicide, described the wish to bring out "the things inside." This poem shocked many members, who understood the description of a dying emotional life. Scenes involving depression and suicide, with associated anger at parents, were played as a result. The importance of communicated felt needs was reviewed.

Predictably, trust of parents, therapists, and others emerged repeatedly, becoming the basis for many scenes. Love also was frequently raised and was related to loneliness, guardedness, and trust. The youngsters' problems with these led the therapists to the decision not to press these issues too closely.

TREATMENT RESULTS: Positive effects for this group were claimed. Eleven out of the sixteen were reported afterwards as largely trouble-free. This included a number of members who participated minimally. Others who participated little stopped coming, and in a later effort, the therapists required a form of payment for entrance into the group. They noted some hesitation about integrating a behavior modification condition into a psychodrama approach, but were pleased when better attendance and involvement resulted.

COMMENTARY: This appears to be an effective intervention for younger adolescents with generally minor offenses. These youngsters were able to remain in the community and could make it to the clinic by themselves. (The issue of family support of this work is not mentioned.) The youngsters were able to accept active techniques, which included pressure on their defenses or emotional "shells." The imposed structure and payment conditions seem to us realistic elements of a program for this population. For older adolescents or more serious offenders, different conditions might be necessary for this program to be accepted. Pay incentives or other privileges might help, and a smaller group might lessen nonparticipation.

SOURCE: Carpenter, P., and Sandberg, S. " 'The Things Inside': Psychodrama with Delinquent Adolescents." *Psychotherapy: Theory, Research and Practice,* 1973, *10*(3), 245-247.

Learning to Negotiate Conflict

AUTHORS: R. E. Kifer, M. A. Lewis, D. R. Green, and E. L. Phillips

PRECIS: Modifying communication processes for better negotiation skills

INTRODUCTION: A common situation for this age group finds the adolescent and a person in authority with opposing wishes. Such conflict situations are especially problematical for delinquents. For most teenagers and their parents, teachers, and so forth, negotiating is all too rarely used at such points. This skill may be absent from the adolescent's repertoire or inconsistent with family communication styles. The authors argue that an educative approach can help develop the ability to negotiate differences between people. Rather than focusing on specific problem behavior, the aim is to teach strategies and stages in the negotiation process. Although therapeutic applicability was not the focus of the paper, teaching interpersonal negotiation skills can be a valuable part of an overall therapeutic plan. For this reason, we have included a summary of the educational steps taken in the project. As always, the reader is advised to consult the original article for more extensive discussion.

TREATMENT METHOD: The project model had three phases; home observation of typical behavior, then training sessions, followed by home observation to assess change. Three adolescents, two female, one male, aged thirteen to seventeen, each with at least one contact with juvenile court, were the subjects. They worked with their parent of the same sex (not an intentional part of the program). On the first home observation visit, the pair were asked to agree on three most difficult problems causing conflict at present. They tried to role play each issue for five minutes to reach a solution. The *training phase,* conducted separately for each pair, employed hypothetical situations for practice, instructions and definitions, and feedback with repeated trials. The training objective was the use of all "negotiation behaviors" in each simulation. These were:

1. *Complete communication*—I state my view, immediately asking for your view or response to mine.

2. *Issue identification*—We say the points where we disagree, calling them "issues," to perhaps lessen the dogmatic nature of the interchange.

3. *Suggestions of options*—Possible answers are offered. Solutions phrased as questions may have a better success rate.

The sequence in training began with a simulation using a hypothetical conflict situation. This was role played for five minutes. Then the same situation was presented, with a list of possible responses and possible consequences. People could add to the list and then discuss which behaviors might have which consequences. They then role played their choices. The child played his or her own role several times and played the parent's role. At a timely point, each pair was told that the training phase would end when all three negotiation behaviors were used in two pretraining discussions. Four to six sessions were needed, lasting seventy-five minutes. Then a final phase repeated the baseline procedure to evaluate progress.

TREATMENT RESULTS: All negotiation behaviors increased in frequency for all parent-child pairs. Home observation showed that negotiation skills had been successfully transferred from the training sessions. Further, the agreements made in posttraining sessions were more frequently kept at home.

COMMENTARY: Several contributors to improved communication were used in this structured procedure. The sequential elements of negotiation were clearly presented. Opportunity to consider means-ends relations was prominent. Being informed of the behaviors needed to terminate training was demonstrated to have a marked positive effect. The use of home observation and telephone contact supported attempts to use the skills outside of the training.

SOURCE: Kifer, R. E., Lewis, M. A., Green, D. R., and Phillips, E. L. "Training Predelinquent Youths and Their Parents to

Negotiate Conflict Situations." *Journal of Applied Behavior Analysis*, 1974, 7, 357-364.

A Program for Parents to Improve Their Children's Communication

AUTHORS: T. V. Lysaght and J. D. Burchard

PRECIS: Changing verbalization patterns of the mother of an antisocial young adolescent

INTRODUCTION: Dysfunctional verbal interactions between mother and child were measured and modified. The authors argue that modifying communication is a foundation for later behavior programs. It may be necessary to deal with family interaction style before other interventions are possible. An example is given in the case of a youngster with multiple difficulties.

CASE HISTORY: Joey was twelve and living in a group home serving boys with learning and behavior problems. Self-care and school performance were poor. He had stopped going to school. His shaky self-image was evident from many self-demeaning statements. Others in the home responded negatively to him, isolating him. (He visited his mother only on weekends.)

TREATMENT METHOD: At the start, pride and confidence were specified as targets for him. He agreed to be the focus in a treatment program. An assignment was a ten-minute discussion on two specific topics at home visits. His mother received a behavior card weekly listing three positive and three negative behaviors of the past week. She also saw an essay he had to write each week for them to discuss. Their discussions were recorded for evaluation purposes.

After baseline data collection, the mother's instructions

were to try to get Joey to talk more about the three appropriate behaviors and to praise him for them. She was to avoid focus on any extensive negative remarks of his, which were usually three times as frequent. The mother got help from the reviewer of the conversation tapes, who called to offer suggestions.

TREATMENT RESULTS: The mother's critical remarks stopped almost immediately, remaining virtually absent through the fifteen weeks of the study. Frequency of praise increased dramatically. It was noted that discussions of the essay (where the mother had not received instructions) continued to show some criticism. Although the authors were primarily concerned to demonstrate modified communication by the mother, they noted that Joey was reported to be greatly improved at his mother's home.

COMMENTARY: The mother's preintervention behavior shows a common pattern of ineffective attempts at verbal control. Extensive review of a teenager's shortcomings is common, even in the face of repeated failure of this approach to have the desired effect. This mother learned two alternatives—praise and withheld criticism (extinction of attention for self-deprecation). The logic of this approach and its demonstrated effect upon the mother make the elements of this program, including homework and tape review, worth considering when the goal is modification of an individual's response pattern.

SOURCE: Lysaght, T. V., and Burchard, J. D. "The Analysis and Modification of a Deviant Parent-Youth Communication Pattern." *Journal of Behavior Therapy and Experimental Psychiatry*, 1975, *6*, 339-342.

Additional Readings

Awad, G. A. "The Early Phase of Psychotherapy with Antisocial Adolescents." *Canadian Journal of Psychiatry,* 1981, *26,* 38-42.

Antisocial behavior of young adolescents, if not a response to transient life stress, reflects serious pathology at an early phase. Youth of this age have distinctive psychic functioning that the therapist should consider. They may be preoccupied with autonomy but not yet ready to grapple with the issue of a separate identity. A therapeutic goal is help for this youngster in achieving a sense of autonomy.

Due to changing moods and situations, the therapists' tasks include empathic listening, interpreting, counseling, educating, and just being a confidant. In early treatment, antisocial youngsters' motivation may be increased by promise of better gratification. This is in contrast to Fraiberg's recommendation, perhaps derived from middle-class neurotic teens, to extend the promise of better ego controls (S. Fraiberg, "Some Considerations in the Introduction to Therapy in Puberty." *Psychoanalytic Study of the Child,* 1955, *10,* 264-286). Other recommendations include a higher activity level by the therapist, willingness to extend oneself (as in involvement with school personnel), making clear the realistic limits of therapeutic help, and avoiding justification or support of antisocial acts.

Fo, W. S. O., and O'Donnell, C. R. "The Buddy System: Relationship and Contingency Conditions in a Community Intervention Program for Youth with Nonprofessionals as Behavior Change Agents." *Journal of Consulting and Clinical Psychology,* 1974, *42,* 163-169.

The authors developed an early intervention program for youngsters (eleven- to seventeen-year-olds who were difficult community management problems) referred from family court. They had histories of truancy, staying out late, fighting, and disruption and poor work in school. "Buddies," aged seventeen to sixty-five, recruited through newspaper ads, were paid modest amounts, ranging up to $144 a month, based on their activity. To earn the full amount, they had to contact each of their three assigned youngsters weekly; submit weekly logs, reports, and behavior data; and attend biweekly training sessions. Training subjects included relationship building, contingency rewards, and targeting behavior problems and goals. This program reduced school truancy; a nonreward buddy relationship had no effect. The addition of behavior rewards up to $10 per month increased gains, such as doing chores at home, observing curfews, and fighting less. No change in school grades was observed. More specific target behaviors, like studying, may need to be taught and reinforced in programs such as this.

Price, C., Price, R. P., and Toomey, B. "The Pre-Delinquent Girl: Does a Volunteer Friend Program Help?" *Adolescence,* 1980, *15*(57), 55-64.

A delinquency prevention program using volunteer "friends" was created to serve the acting-out female at risk. Most of the girls were adolescents, although the entire age range served was six to twenty-two. Girls were referred by courts, schools, and agencies. The girls' participation was voluntary. The plan was to present each girl with a corrective model, to demonstrate community concern, and to give them a better example of how one copes with problems. An extensive evaluation of the project was done. Feedback from all sources indicated a positive effect on most girls. The girls liked their volunteers and valued the program highly, although they reported relatively little help with solutions of explicit problems. Future prevention programs may usefully incorporate more problem-solving assistance for the girls, such as referral by the volunteers to discussion groups or professional help.

Stuart, R. B., Jayaratne, S., and Tripodi, T. "Changing Adolescent Deviant Behaviour Through Reprogramming the Behaviour of Parents and Teachers: An Experimental Evaluation." *Canadian Journal of Behavioural Science,* 1976, *8*(2), 132-144.

A single technique, a behavior contract with home-based reinforcement of improved school behaviors, was used, with some positive results. Referral was through school authorities. The implementation of the contract alone resulted in change, without requiring direct modification of communication or family decision-making methods. A therapist worked with parents and teachers to obtain positively stated goals and potential reinforcers. Responsibilities of the referred adolescent were worked out, and a three-column contract was completed. For each behavior, privileges desired, responsibilities, and, wherever possible, bonuses or sanctions were clearly described. Family sessions were to examine and improve contracts. Contact was for up to four months. Several modest gains were noted, including teacher and counselor evaluation and maternal perception of a better relationship.

Unkovic, C. M., Brown, W. R., and Mierswa, C. G. "Counter-attack on Juvenile Delinquency: A Configurational Approach." *Adolescence*, 1978, *13*(51), 401-410.

A special camping program for predelinquent, delinquent, and school-expelled fourteen- to seventeen-year-olds is described. Developed by an air force community action group, the program has several notable goals and features. The campers are 90 percent problem youths and 10 percent achieving youths. The better functioning boys are not labeled as models—labels are avoided for all. Counselors do not reveal their back-home occupations (policemen, graduate students in several fields) until the very end. Counselors receive instructions in establishing rapport. A sixteen-hour schedule includes vocational demonstrations and self-care instruction. Evaluation showed improved behavior and self-esteem. Although control figures are lacking, recidivism appears to be low.

Vogt, A. T. "The Motorcycle as a Psychological Tool." *Psychological Reports*, 1977, *40*, 9-10.

This article suggests treatment opportunities in guided group activities for poorly socialized predelinquents. A club for minibikers aged twelve to fifteen had many members who had been in juvenile court. Several activities in the club promoted improved adjustment in these boys and girls. These included need for maintenance, safety, and concern and respect for others' property. The more poorly adjusted youngsters ignored these behaviors, ignoring maintenance, running into others, and stealing parts. Group feedback was swift to such actions, and sharp changes in attitude and behavior were noted after accidents or bike failures. Earned membership and positive peer pressure were two important helpful features. Reports of these youngsters' school problems and domestic violence lessened, and pride in achievement began to be noted.

Delinquency

"Delinquency" connotes a wide range of antisocial acts. Adolescents labeled delinquents are at serious risk of being institutionalized or jailed or have been so already. Legal use of the term can be confusing. Malmquist lists six antisocial categories that contain the word delinquent (C. P. Malmquist, Handbook of Adolescence, *New York: Jason Aronson, 1978).*

Whereas prevention was of prominent concern in the previous section, it is absent here. The major emphasis is on rehabilitation of the institutionalized delinquent. Traditional psychotherapy has rarely been considered effective. Multifaceted approaches take advantage of environmental, legal, and peer group pressures in developing residential programs. Some interesting attempts to modify maladaptive cognitions have been explored. Several articles delineate specific behavior problems in this population. The hope is that by increasing prosocial competence, alternate behaviors can be encouraged to improve the youngster's postplacement chances. The extent of delinquency in our society and the largely disappointing results of most treatment efforts to date make further treatment development essential.

245

Increasing Involvement of Male
Offenders in Treatment

AUTHOR: R. L. Schwitzgebel

PRECIS: Introduction and gradual shifts of reinforcers for attendance to assist relationship formation

INTRODUCTION: This article may be especially important for therapists working with committed or other involuntary patients. Schwitzgebel's goal was to provide a strategy for beginning a therapeutic relationship, including regular attendance at sessions, with adolescents showing serious delinquent patterns. Diagnosed as psychopathic, borderline, or the like, with police records, they rarely seek help. Subculture opinion that one is weak or crazy to seek a therapist is another source of resistance. If a delinquent does manage to keep an appointment and has awkward interchanges with a therapist who waits for verbal interchanges, he may see no purpose in returning.

Several writers' views on beginning treatment with delinquents have some elements in common. Surprising, unexpected behavior, such as an active manner or telling jokes, helps to ease the anxiety surrounding entry into the therapy process. The therapist should avoid those awkward periods of waiting for the patient's verbal initiative. The therapist's activity gives clues to what is expected. Without such clues, the minimally socialized young patient may leave to avoid anxiety.

TREATMENT METHOD: Some of the adolescents in this study had previously refused treatment. A third had been imprisoned for eighteen months on average. They were sought on the streets or at amusement places. They were told they could earn $1 an hour giving interviews and would be taped. A requirement for eligibility was a court record. The first interview, if accepted, took place in a local fast-food place ("home territory"). After talking for long enough to earn some money, they had to go to the office, where payment was made and a second appointment was arranged for the next day (rapid follow-up).

At subsequent sessions, one experimental group received reinforcements (casual giving of cigarettes, candy, or cash) for arrival on time. Another group received them based on other socially appropriate behaviors. The first group's lateness was somewhat less than that of the second.

TREATMENT RESULTS: The boys seemed to look forward to the interviews eventually. They felt challenged and became involved. After fifteen to twenty-five sessions, reinforcers were gradually decreased to zero, with attendance and promptness remaining unchanged.

COMMENTARY: Some aspects of the therapy process clearly became reinforcers because these youngsters continued to attend. Although the author's view argues that the reinforcers are therapist behavior, we would suggest the additional reinforcing properties of relationship formation, behavior change, and gaining of insight as possibilities. The clinic staff used this procedure with considerable success, except in cases of serious narcotic abusers. This is a useful technique for a traditionally reluctant subgroup.

SOURCE: Schwitzgebel, R. L. "Preliminary Socialization for Psychotherapy of Behavior-Disordered Adolescents." *Journal of Consulting and Clinical Psychology,* 1969, *33,* 71-77.

Training of Tendency to Give Positive Verbal Feedback

AUTHORS: J. G. Emshoff, W. H. Redd, and W. S. Davidson

PRECIS: Achieving generalization of prosocial verbalizations

INTRODUCTION: Teaching positive social behavior to delinquents has been shown to be feasible and worthwhile. Efforts to promote the use of these new skills in places outside the learning situation, however, often bring little result ("poor generalization of effect"). A common view is that the stimulus conditions that would result in the new behavior are too narrowly presented. The authors' modification in procedure is to treat generalization problems much earlier in the process when teaching prosocial behavior to delinquents. From the beginning, the new behaviors are presented as desirable in many situations.

TREATMENT METHOD: Four residents in a home for adolescents with delinquent and psychiatric problems were involved. All were observed to rarely make positive verbal comments to others. In thirty-minute training sessions, each youngster received one point and verbal praise for making audible and situation-appropriate positive remarks to another. Each point was worth three cents. Seven thirty-minute training sessions were held over a two-week period. For two of the teenagers, training was held at different times and places, during different activities, not always with the same trainer. Their learning environments were thus more varied than for the others, for whom the conditions were the same for all sessions.

TREATMENT RESULTS: All the teenagers made ten to fifty times more positive comments in the training sessions. Those trained in varying places with different trainers doubled their rate of positive comments outside the training sessions and maintained part of that increase for at least three weeks after training was over and no more money was given. Such positive gains were not clear for the two adolescents in the constant-training situation. The conclusion is that for those exposed to varied trial conditions, there were reinforcers besides points, money, and praise at work.

COMMENTARY: The major achievement of this work is the method of increasing positive behavior where the training rewards are not present. It is clear that the procedure that featured an early variety of places and activities provided a more fruitful training experience. This was presented as a research study, but several issues for adolescent treatment can be raised. Delinquents and disturbed adolescents who have rarely done so are able to use positive comment. To be incorporated into a treatment program, a longer training program would probably be advisable. The amount of reward could be decreased gradually (fading) as the behavior appears to become a stable new part of the behavior repertoire. A goal of such a program is that new reinforcers, such as people's responses and increased feelings of self-regard, would help maintain this behavior. Regular interviews with the adolescent could help him examine the benefits of this new learning.

SOURCE: Emshoff, J. G., Redd, W. H., and Davidson, W. S. "Generalization Training and the Transfer of Prosocial Behavior in Delinquent Adolescents." *Journal of Behavior Therapy and Experimental Psychiatry,* 1976, *7,* 141-144.

Treating Impulsivity and Program Noncompliance with Self-Instruction

AUTHORS: J. J. Snyder and M. J. White

PRECIS: Cognitive self-instruction techniques as a necessary addition to an operant treatment program

INTRODUCTION: For delinquents in a controlled setting, a point system or similar control system is not sufficient. Snyder and White offered a method of achieving self-control of behaviors to institutionalized adolescents who were not responding to the program's reward and punishment system. The adolescents were told of this serious problem and placed in a cognitive self-instruction training group to examine their response style and work on alternatives. The authors stressed the necessity for a plan for developing internal controls, even in a program emphasizing controls and discipline by external authorities.

TREATMENT METHOD: These adolescents had been placed in this residential setting, whose philosophy was based on the Achievement Place model. Their problem behaviors ranged from major family conflict to theft and drug abuse. They were chosen because of their minimal response to the behavior controls imposed by the program. The overall behavior goal was increased involvement in the program. Target behaviors selected were increased class attendance, improved self-care and carrying out of tasks, and reduced impulsive behavior. The working definition of each target was spelled out to the adolescent.

The adolescents were fifteen minority youngsters aged fourteen to seventeen, both sexes. They included blacks, Hispanics, and whites. They were randomly assigned to three groups, one of which was an untreated control group. Cognitive self-instruction was one of the two treatments attempted (the other, known as contingency awareness, showed little result and will not be summarized). The adolescent was seen privately, and examples of his major difficulties, such as getting up in the morning, were discussed. Each youngster was taught the concept of private speech and how people use it to guide and correct their behavior. In groups, a likely private verbalization for unwanted behavior was suggested. Thus, for a *situation,* being told to arise, a private *verbalization* might be, "No way. I like it where I am." This would be followed by the *behavior* of not getting up, with the *consequence* of loss of points. Therapists used modeling, role playing, and social reinforcement to construct the four-step sequences of situation, verbalization, behavior, and consequence for each member. Using the same techniques, the group explored how self-defeating the sequence was and developed possible alternative verbalizations: "It feels nice here, but I'll lose points, which means no cigarettes. Let me start by opening my eyes. . . ." An alternative sequence of *behavior* (getting up) and *consequence* (getting points) was accomplished. The adolescents rehearsed these changing words and reactions actively, thus making the sequences more "their own." Adolescents role played staff and helped each other improve their own verbalizing ability. Group reinforcement of success was a highly valued part of this process. The therapists saw a need for protection of the teenagers from their overreaction to failure incidents. They helped the youngsters to learn coping statements, such as, "I blew this, but I can make a mistake and still try. I don't have to be perfect, just better."

TREATMENT RESULTS: This treatment group was the only one of the three to achieve behavior gains, which were maintained at a six-week follow-up. Class attendance increased, observers' ratings showed fewer impulsive incidents, and responsibilities were more frequently met. The data suggest that the point system by itself was only slightly helpful but that the verbal self-instruction intervention led to much greater compliance with the institutional program.

COMMENTARY: This work provides support for the effectiveness of tailored verbal techniques for the delinquent. The common view of the nonverbally oriented adolescent as unresponsive to verbal intervention is increasingly under challenge. This work is one of the significant number offering planned specific interventions based on analysis of the youngsters' conceptual or behavior deficiencies. A notable feature was the introduction of the program to the adolescent, clarifying, at the outset, the predicament of having no dependable self-control. Though this work was part of an experiment, its clinical implications are worth review when planning an individual comprehensive treatment plan for the delinquent. The six-week follow-up data is welcome. In institutions, however, the culture may erode gains; thus we suggest an even longer follow-up evaluation.

SOURCE: Snyder, J. J., and White, M. J. "The Use of Cognitive Self-Instruction in the Treatment of Behaviorally Disturbed Adolescents." *Behavior Therapy*, 1979, *10*, 227-235.

Treating Low Self-Esteem in
Delinquent Females

AUTHORS: J. P. Reardon and D. J. Tosi

PRECIS: Structured relaxation and rational imagery techniques
to assist development of feelings of competence

INTRODUCTION: Low self-esteem, related to inability to cope
with external demands, may develop as a major problem in antisocial adolescents. Repeated failures may reinforce misconcep-
tions, making subsequent attempts more stressful. In some people this leads to an avoidance pattern, but in delinquents acting
out is more prevalent. The goal here was to raise self-esteem in a
group of institutionalized delinquent girls using Tosi's method
of rational stage directed imagery (RSDI).

TREATMENT METHOD: The theory of this treatment assumed
six stages comprised the change process: *awareness*—an introduction to new options, contradictions in one's assumptions, an
orientation to change; *exploration*—early attempts at new options, the co-beginning of cognitive restructuring and resistance;
commitment to rational/constructive action—developing deeper
insights and new reactions, producing a conflict about change;
implementation—increased, postcommitment use of new skills;
internalization—greater proficiency reflecting conflict-free use
of adaptive skills; and *change and redirection*—acknowledging
change and independent use of skills.
      During the first three of these, deep relaxation was intro-
duced. Basic ideas of rational-emotive therapy were briefly explained (A. Ellis, *Reason and Emotion in Psychotherapy,* New
York: Lyle Stuart, 1962). Each teenager identified an emotionally upsetting situation. She closed her eyes, visualized the
event, and recalled her feelings. She was helped to challenge the
irrational thoughts about that time. Rational self-talk and development of better understanding and paths of action completed the sequence.
      This sequence—relaxation, visualization, reaction, challenge,

review of rational alternatives with self-talk, and imagining improved outcomes and feelings—was used in two ways. It was used with the girls' reported upsetting problems and with scenes the authors designed to evoke predictably problematic scenes.

Therapists assisted the girls through the developmental stages, allowing each to work at her own pace. They provided praise for completion of each sequence. Homework, consisting of *in vivo* tasks, was assigned at each session. The rational sequence was to be imagined and employed for assigned problems.

TREATMENT RESULTS: There were notable increases in measured self-esteem, which were maintained at two-month posttraining. Examination of posttraining self-esteem suggests several sources of gain for the delinquent girls. They no longer saw themselves as equal in "badness" to their criminal acts. It was possible to think more hopefully about oneself as well. The girls were less negative about society and about their ability to interact with the world. Depression had lifted somewhat and improvement continued after training had ended. These gains were significant when compared with a group receiving a "rational restructuring" program (which omitted relaxation and the stages of development).

COMMENTARY: The use of imagery techniques has received increasing attention recently. The work described here used imagery with a group usually resistant to verbal intervention. This population was quite receptive, however, to relaxation and emotionally provoking stimulus material in a guided, structured sequence. The extending of imagery techniques to other specific problems, possibly with relaxation and within a structured program, warrants consideration.

SOURCE: Reardon, J. P., and Tosi, D. J. "The Effects of Rational Stage Directed Imagery on Self-Concept and Reduction of Psychological Stress in Adolescent Delinquent Females." *Journal of Clinical Psychology*, 1977, *33*(4), 1084-1092.

A Cognitive Approach to Group
Therapy for Delinquents

AUTHOR: H. Harari

PRECIS: Guidelines for cognitive therapy

INTRODUCTION: Traditional "cathartic" therapies have not been notably successful with delinquent adolescents. Harari, a social psychologist, uses Fritz Heider's balance theory to show why certain therapy approaches are better received by this population. He rejects a primarily cathartic group approach and describes a group program stressing the importance of certain cognitive variables. Judgments one makes of others' actions influence like or dislike of them, and people have styles of judging. They attribute friendly or unfriendly motives to others' actions. If an enemy does something you like, however, there is a "cognitive imbalance." This can be resolved, among other ways, by deciding to dislike the enemy less or attributing negative motives for his or her actions. If a boy does not expect help, but sees the therapist as powerful, there is a cognitive imbalance. According to Harari's research, people manifest different styles of restoring balance. They may change their view of the person or reinterpret his or her behavior. Imbalances exist in needy youngsters who see the therapist as lacking the power to help. It is essential to explore and modify these imbalances before therapy effects can be expected. Harari discusses ways to do this with delinquents, who usually present with little experience at thinking through such problems.

CASE HISTORY: Phil was fifteen and in treatment by court mandate, still insisting he needed no help. He was described as somewhat hysterical. The Heider category that bothered him the most turned out to be Type VII (see "Treatment Method"). His resolution of the hypothetical situations of this type was to *deny* that B had done anything (changing to a Type IV situation).

Other important information about Phil was obtained from the Gordon Survey of Interpersonal Values. He scored high in recognition seeking, which is consistent with denying credit to others. Phil disliked the group, which tried to help. He wanted no help and sneered at people's remarks. As a high recognition seeker, he found a way to like the group—by claiming it was offering him no help.

TREATMENT METHOD: An early step in the group meetings is to assess people's needs and expectations. For those who expect help, a more directive approach is advised at the outset. Failure to respond to the neediness usually brings poor results. The therapist should establish an expectation in the group that he or she will be an active respondent.

In assessing needs and expectations, questioning at first should be direct, although the therapist should expect limited results. One should avoid confrontation at this stage. A more structured way is to present examples of Heider's eight interpersonal situation categories and getting reactions. These categories are:

Type I. A likes B, who is doing what A likes.
Type II. A likes B, who is not doing what A dislikes.
Type III. A *dislikes* B, who is doing what A dislikes.
Type IV. A *dislikes* B, who is not doing what A likes.

Type V. A likes B, who does what A dislikes.
Type VI. A likes B, who doesn't do what A likes.
Type VII. A *dislikes* B, who does what A likes.
Type VIII. A *dislikes* B, who doesn't do what A dislikes.

The first four are considered balanced, the last four imbalanced. Type I is considered the best solution. As they are presented with hypothetical situations of each type, adolescents' preferred patterns can be made clear. The consequences of their ways of resolving unbalanced cognitions are clarified in the group discussions.

TREATMENT RESULTS: Phil's Type II solution resulted in his relaxing in the group and becoming able to discuss his problems. He was eventually able to overcome his strongly held attitude and admit the group was helpful. He had arrived at a Type I resolution. He worked much more successfully in the group and terminated after seven months of group treatment.

COMMENTARY: This system offers a novel diagnostic and prescriptive framework for a difficult subgroup of adolescents. The interested reader will need to read the full article and other work by Harari and Heider. This work is helpful in showing the range of cognitive adaptation in delinquents and their differing treatment needs in a group. We must remember that although delinquents are a category in society, this label is not a diagnosis. Individual behavior strengths and deficits in these youngsters still require clarification as a prelude to treatment.

Harari is one of many who advise therapists to be more assertive, clarifying their own roles and exploring their patient's expectations of the group. We suggest that this is especially necessary for poorly motivated adolescents.

SOURCE: Harari, H. "Cognitive Manipulations with Delinquent Adolescents in Group Therapy." *Psychotherapy: Theory, Research and Practice,* 1972, *9*(4), 303-307.

See also Harari, H. "Interpersonal Models in Psychotherapy and Counseling: A Social-Psychological Analysis of a Clinical Problem." *Journal of Abnormal Psychology,* 1971, *78,* 127-133.

Heider, F. *The Psychology of Interpersonal Relations.* New York: Wiley, 1958.

A Group Training Model for Impulsive Unsocialized Delinquents

AUTHOR: J. C. Westman

PRECIS: A training experience emphasizing authority, limit setting, and control issues in long-term treatment

INTRODUCTION: Antisocial adolescents are considered patients, not prisoners, in this hospital adolescent unit. Traditional group methods are less successful with adolescents, still less so with teens with major behavior or social deficits. Limit testing, poor impulse control, and reluctance to think about problems are some reasons for this. The author describes a modified group designed for this population.

TREATMENT METHOD: The group addressed itself to several concerns. One was problems in group membership versus narcissistic self-involvement. Attractions of the group were enhanced to make membership more desirable. Peer pressure to act in ways to stay in the group were thus more effective. Desirable features were avoidance of a disliked activity taking place at the same time, a waiting period to get into the group, refreshment, and new gossip. A second concern was problems of identification with adult models. Instead of a friendly relationship-building approach, likely to be rejected, the intent was to gain the group's respect during the give-and-take, or testing, phase at the outset. The therapist became a model for identification and imitation by able and consistent responding to the provocations posed by teenagers searching for signs of weakness or sensitivity. A third concern was poor understanding of conventional behavior and realistic limits. Problem areas included unrealistic notions about authority figures, ignorance about conventional behaviors, and how to enjoy themselves in socially acceptable ways. The therapists explored with them what was considered sick or normal. Peers were encouraged to point out realities because their comments often had more impact than those of the therapist. A fourth concern was problems of impulse control and nonresponse to verbal mediation and therapy. Staff dealt with this by imposing rules. Members must sit around the table, and acting out would lead to early dismissal from the session. No side conversations, no moving around, no activity other than the complete freedom to talk about anything of general interest were the prevailing rules. External control by rules, especially at the outset, was clearly more effective than verbal therapy. Support for this approach was demonstrated within a month, when behavior control was exercised mostly by peers. A fifth concern was difficulty in placing oneself in a context. With concrete, self-related thinking, largely related to immediate needs, these youngsters had not come to see themselves as patients or to develop motivation for change. Talk was used to conceal or as exhibitionistic behavior, with any "insights" being shallow. Intervention was based more on nonverbal behaviors and issues, which were raised tentatively or tangentially. Discussions were sometimes kept on a hypothetical basis or were about others outside of the group. This was especially helpful in anxious discussions about girls.

TREATMENT RESULT: For the first month of the year-long period described, direct control was required until the boys accepted the failure of their manipulative efforts. Pro-staff comments were rarely genuine and usually intended to dislodge an unsuccessful antistaff leader. Peer control of most negative behaviors was achieved by the third month. Attitudes toward the male therapist remained hostile for several more months. After they diminished, the group sought direction from him, especially concerning problems of discharge. The presence of a female (nurse) observer throughout the group stimulated their fantasies about male-female collaboration and the effects of women on their own behavior.

COMMENTARY: The chief contribution of this work is the analysis of major behavior weaknesses and prescriptive guidelines for assisting their correction. There is a focus upon intrapsychic as well as behavior change. The five areas listed represent practical translation of a psychodynamic perspective into specific treatment issues. These ideas would in all probability apply to adolescents in residential treatment and community group homes as well as hospitals.

SOURCE: Westman, J. C. "Group Psychotherapy with Hospitalized Delinquent Adolescents." *International Journal of Group Psychotherapy*, 1961, *11*, 410-418.

Additional Readings

Chwast, J. "Control: The Key to Offender Treatment." *American Journal of Psychotherapy*, 1965, *19*, 116-125.

In treating delinquents, strong external control is vital, but it must be skillfully used, based on an assessment of the individual's status. Four arenas of control are distinguished—of social structures, of the social process (arrest, trial, and so forth), of outcome (reduction of delinquent behavior), where most therapy effort is placed, and of self-developed inner controls, a desirable but usually distant goal. Therapeutic method involves strong external control, while the individual therapist discusses problems, offers advice, and works toward the beginning of attempts at internal controls. The therapist will need to be comfortable with manipulating external controls, as needed. By themselves, management of social structures and process and individual therapy are known to be largely ineffective. Used together, they are a complex but more effective treatment approach.

Chwast, J. "Principles and Techniques of Offender Therapy." In J. Masserman (Ed.), *Current Psychiatric Therapies*, Vol. 6. New York: Grune and Stratton, 1966.

Several guidelines for treatment of the unmotivated offender are discussed. This work is derived from experience in the clinic of the Association for the Psychiatric Treatment of Offenders. The work of Melitta Schmideberg is acknowledged.

(Also see the *Journal of Offender Therapy*.) External controls, including court threats, must be strong at the outset. Acceptance of the patient is shown by demonstrating understanding of his or her communications while avoiding a permissive, sympathetic response style. Goals at this point should be reality based and limited, with concrete, specific suggestions being frequently necessary. Crises and regressions are predictable. Insight is experienced as upsetting. The therapist can make little use of the transference relationship and should not encourage its development. Interpretations, if tentative and partial, may be less threatening. Comments that increase guilt will not necessarily produce acting out—they should be tried. The therapist should keep in mind that this patient typically withholds information and tries to get people to act on a distorted story. A variety of positive supporting activities may be tried, including advice on building on new skills and assisting reliance upon several helping agencies rather than on the therapist only.

Didato, S. V. "Delinquents in Group Therapy: Some New Techniques." *Adolescence,* 1970, *5*(18), 207-222.

A therapy group for delinquents was developed with four primary goals: ability to experience stronger affects, expressing them verbally without inappropriate action; greater empathic capacity; greater identification with the therapist; and more verbal resolution of intragroup conflicts. The sessions were structured and employed fantasy and imagery techniques and probe questions to get reports of personal feelings. The boys attempted to set up their own structures to judge their peers' behavior. Didato suggests that therapists need a high tolerance for anxiety and must actively reach out to develop and maintain contact. Also important is the therapist's effort to maintain a stance of more objective involvement, bearing in mind the considerable pressures and emotions evoked in attempts to work with this population.

Evans, J. "Analytic Group Therapy with Delinquents." *Adolescence,* 1966, *1*, 180-196.

When a boy is selected for therapy in this residential program for delinquents, attendance is mandatory. This requirement is made because the inevitable hostility to and resentment of treatment is better dealt with by expression within therapy rather than outside. Derived from a Tavistock group approach, this model stresses attention to the group process, including clarification of feelings, motivations, fears, and defenses. Interpretations are made to the group—it has been found that focus on only a single person may lead to general inattention. Little direct advice is given here, the therapist reminding people that advice is available in many other places in the institution.

The process of an illustrative session showed the boys were able to discuss, albeit indirectly, strongly felt issues. Although silence was a predominant response to the therapist's interventions, the ensuing themes suggested that there was reluctant listening to him. Extreme rapid mood and opinion swings were the norm. Informal evaluation suggested better subsequent control over aggression and ability to look differently at problems and to handle more anxiety.

Sanson-Fisher, R. W., Seymour, F. W., and Baer, D. M. "Training Staff to Alter Delinquents' Conversation." *Journal of Behavior Therapy and Experimental Psychiatry*, 1976, *7*, 243-247.

The authors speculate that peer culture, rather than staff culture, is the best focus of consistent intervention effort. They found that training staff to respond in a consistent way (positive attention to positive comments) was insufficient to produce noticeable change, other than when the reinforcing staff were present. However, a longer trial period than the one used here (five days) might in our opinion be capable of producing better results.

Schwartz, L. J. "Treatment of the Adolescent Psychopath—Theory and Case Report." *Psychotherapy: Theory, Research and Practice*, 1967, *4*(3), 133-137.

Schwartz writes that successful individual therapy with psychopathic adolescents requires two factors. One is a close, sensitive therapy relationship, gained by investigating the patient's narcissistic and environmental needs. The second is assistance of delay of gratification, which is necessary before the patient can examine his or her needs and reactions to failure or success.

In early sessions with an eighteen-year-old female, Schwartz discussed her plans for deceptions and parental rule violations, even suggesting additions to her methods. He encouraged more complex strategies, which increased ability to delay. The relationship became stronger, based partly on therapist praise of her strategies, until delay was easier and therapist approval seemed more sought than the original desired objects.

She showed some identification with the therapist, becoming interested in helping her friends, until it could be shown that she could give advice, but not follow it herself. After some self-control was demonstrated, the relationship between anger at her world and resultant self-defeating acts was explored. This was occasionally followed by rageful outbursts transferred toward the therapist, who was not assisting psychopathic behavior. An underlying dynamic now emerged. If she succeeded in a manipulation, she felt ungratified because her environment was shown to be powerless. If she got caught or failed, she felt rageful and rejected. Regular discussion of her efforts and relation to her past in the style of traditional psychotherapy could begin at this point.

Shoemaker, M. E. "Group Assertion Training for Institutionalized Male Delinquents." In J. L. Stumphauzer (Ed.). *Progress in Behavior Therapy with Delinquents.* Springfield, Ill.: Thomas, 1979.

The author describes several benefits of assertiveness training for delinquents. They can learn a more appropriate and successful method of gaining objectives, which also avoids violations of others' rights and personal space. A subgroup of delinquents, aged thirteen to sixteen, in residential treatment, noted to be passive and withdrawn, seemed an appropriate target group. After two weeks of nondirected discussion, a system of token payments for assertion was initiated. Reinforced behaviors were expression of feelings, thoughts, and problems and attempts at solutions. The boys were taught the distinction between assertive behavior, labeled a "claim," and other, less-advised options, like walking away or aggression. Generalization was helped by assignments to keep records of "claims" made during the week. The program was revised, expanded, and given the name "Mental Kung Fu," taking advantage of current interest in the martial arts. A points-level system with group meetings and tokens was used. Assertive behavior was increased; aggression showed a moderate decrease. For future work, the author advises eight- to twelve-week groups and thorough staff training.

Stuart, R. B., and Lott, L. A. "Behavioral Contracting with Delinquents: A Cautionary Note." *Journal of Behavior Therapy and Experimental Psychiatry,* 1972, *3,* 161-169.

These authors suggest that success in contracting is primarily a function of therapist skill in mediating, that is, managing conflict during the developing of agreements. They reviewed treatment of ninety-four delinquent or predelinquent adolescents with their families. Neither characteristics of patients (such as age, race, or family income) nor treatment variables (number of contracts) predicted better outcome. Two important aspects of conflict resolution are cited here. First, the therapist as mediator should take advantage of pressure generated by the crisis situation or court referral; this assists the parties to agree to conditions they would otherwise resist. Second, all parties must be helped to avoid loss of face. This contract can be maintained only with further effort, incompatible with a sense of defeat in negotiation. Skill is needed to remind the bargainers that the agreement represents a gain for each side.

5 ◎◎◎◎◎◎◎◎◎◎◎◎◎◎◎◎◎◎

Sexual Problems

◎◎◎◎◎◎◎◎◎◎◎◎◎◎◎◎◎◎

Rapid increase in sexual maturation is a defining feature of the adolescent period. A major task of adolescent development is the integration of resulting sexual fantasies and behaviors with personal values and societal expectations. This occurs gradually throughout adolescence and parallels social and intellectual maturation.

Each individual arrives at adolescence with gender identity (sense of being a male or female) well established. Only rarely is there a lack of congruence between gender identity and physical anatomy, but when this occurs, it can lead to serious adjustment difficulties (L. M. Lothstein, "The Adolescent Gender Dysphoric Patient: An Approach to Treatment and Management," *Journal of Pediatric Psychology*, 1980, 5, 93-109). Persistent dissatisfaction with one's own anatomical sex and a wish to have different genitals and live as a member of the opposite sex is diagnostic for transsexualism (American Psychiatric Association, *Diagnostic and Statistical Manual*, 3rd ed., Washington, D.C.: American Psychiatric Association, 1980). Until fairly recently, this condition was seen as irreversible and the transsexual had to make whatever adjustment he or she could to a profoundly unsettling situation. Currently, there are several treatment options, each of which is described in this chapter.

Sexual preference is much less clearly determined at the beginning of adolescence than is gender identity. Constitutional factors and early experiences within the family may predispose one toward either homosexual or heterosexual orientation, but chance factors, such as the availability of heterosexual partners or seduction by an older homosexual, also exert an influence on ultimate outcome (A. Freud, *Normality and Pathology in Childhood*, New York: International Universities Press, 1965). Whatever the outcome, its congruence with self-image, personal values, and family and societal expectations will be important factors in whether or not an individual seeks psychological treatment for homosexuality.

Other sexual problems that bring adolescents into treatment include exhibitionism, voyeurism, and the commission of acts of sexual violence. All of these result in conflict with societal codes and laws, and treatment often occurs under duress or out of fear that legal sanctions will be imposed.

Victims of sexual violence or abuse also have an acute need for psychological treatment. Without appropriate crisis intervention and follow-up treatment, they are likely to sustain long-term, debilitating psychological complications.

Strictly speaking, teenage pregnancy is not a psychological disorder, but it is responsible for a variety of physical and psychological complications for the mother-to-be and her offspring. Those who become pregnant as teenagers are more likely to have pregnancy and birth complications and to have offspring at risk for developmental disorders; they are less likely to complete school or to achieve economic independence (P. R. Magrab, and J. Danielson-Murphy, "Adolescent Pregnancy: A Re-

view," *Journal of Clinical Child Psychology,* 1979, *8,* 121-125).
Preventing unwanted pregnancies in adolescence has numerous
benefits, both for the individuals involved and for society.

A variety of treatment strategies has been used to deal
with problems of adolescent sexual development. Social skills
deficits are present with almost all manifestations of sexual
problems, and social skills training is an important component
of most successful treatment programs. Such specific treatment
techniques as desensitization, operant reinforcement, and aversive training have all been used to good effect, and individual,
group, and family modalities have a place in treatment planning. Specific treatments should take place within the context
of an ongoing therapeutic relationship. Past sexual history, current motivational conflicts, and family and peer group supports
and pressures should all be carefully explored. Long-term follow-
up is an essential part of treatment.

Gender Identity Disorders

Gender identity disorder of childhood has its origins in earliest childhood experience and is usually first manifest in the preschool years. Dissatisfaction with sexual anatomy and sex role assignment, insistence that one is really a member of the opposite sex, cross dressing, and preference for activities typically associated with the opposite sex are all signs of gender identity disorder. Many children with this problem adopt a homosexual orientation in adolescence; a few continue to manifest gender identity disorder in the form of transsexualism (American Psychiatric Association, Diagnostic and Statistical Manual, *3rd ed., Washington, D.C.: American Psychiatric Association, 1980). Transsexualism occurs only rarely, but in some cases the dissatisfaction with sexual anatomy is so profound as to lead to requests for sex reassignment surgery. Until recent years there has been no effective treatment, but now surgery and gender identity change are both treatment options.*

Family Treatment for Gender Disturbed Boys

AUTHORS: J. E. Bates, W. M. Skilbeck, K. V. R. Smith, and P. M. Bentler

PRECIS: A family oriented treatment program to change behaviors reflective of gender disturbance

INTRODUCTION: In the preadolescent boy, gender disturbance can be manifest in a variety of ways, including preference for female toys and activities, feminine mannerisms, and crossdressing. Often there is a high degree of family conflict about such behaviors; and as time passes, many of these children become isolated from peer group relationships. Bates and his colleagues have developed an early intervention program to modify feminine behaviors before they lead to more serious social and sexual adjustment difficulties.

The families of twenty boys presenting with gender disturbed behavior were invited to participate in a treatment program, and sixteen accepted. Children ranged in age from five to thirteen. Families were heterogeneous in terms of socioeconomic level and cultural background.

TREATMENT METHOD: In the beginning there were three main treatment components. The first was evaluation, consisting of parent interviews focused on psychosocial history and current family dynamics and child play interviews directed toward observing play preferences and eliciting information about family and peer relationships. The second component involved play therapy sessions in which masculine behaviors and interests were systematically rewarded. The third involved parent meetings to explore parents' feelings about the child's behavior and to teach them behavior modification principles and strategies.

As treatment progressed, it became apparent that many of the boys were deficient in social skills independent of gender disturbance. They resisted parental authority, failed to carry out family responsibilities, fought with their siblings, were bossy in relation to their peers, insisted on having their own way, and showed poor sportsmanship in competitive games. As a response to these deficiencies, social skills training groups were developed. Male cotherapists who ran the groups developed individualized goals for each child. For one it might be increasing assertiveness, for another, decreasing aggressiveness, and for still another, becoming more actively involved in ongoing activities. Goals were discussed at the beginning of each session and points were given for progress. Extra points were earned when all group members made good progress, and points could be exchanged for money.

During the boys' group meetings, parents also met in groups. Male and female cotherapists who led the groups helped them to discuss openly their feelings about their sons' behavior. Fathers were assisted in planning father-son activities, and both parents were encouraged to cooperate in promoting such activities. Behavior modification strategies were taught and specific applications were discussed. As an offshoot of group meetings, a fathers' and sons' group that met every other week to engage in planned activities like bowling and miniature golf was formed.

TREATMENT RESULTS: The general impression among clinical staff was one of improved social skills and increased masculine interests. Verbal reports from parents and children indicated more play with same-sex peers, better peer relationships, more interest in masculine play, and decreased cross-dressing, doll play, and feminine imitation. Follow-up questionnaire responses at one and a half years indicated general behavioral improvement, increased masculinity, and improved social relationships.

COMMENTARY: This program represents a multimodal attack on a multifaceted problem of development. Without changes in their parents' attitudes and behaviors, boys who have learned to be more masculine would not be rewarded for this at home; and without improved social skills, they would not get the opportunity to try out new behaviors in natural peer group settings.

More evaluation is needed to document specific behavioral changes, but this program defines an approach that can be used clinically and can be refined in response to further research data.

SOURCE: Bates, J. E., Skilbeck, W. M., Smith, K. V. R., and Bentler, P. M. "Intervention with Families of Gender Disturbed Boys." *American Journal of Orthopsychiatry*, 1975, *45*, 150-157.

Inpatient Treatment

AUTHORS: C. W. Davenport and S. I. Harrison

PRECIS: Successful gender identity change in a female adolescent transsexual

INTRODUCTION: The literature on successful postpubertal change in sexual identity is limited. Davenport and Harrison report on a fourteen-year-old girl treated on an inpatient basis for twenty months following a request for a sex change operation.

CASE HISTORY: The patient was the second child in a family of four children. The oldest was a boy, and she was the oldest of the three girls. The father presented himself as a patient and long-suffering man who cared for his family, and the mother presented as tense and insecure, revealing a long history of depression. As a young child, the patient had been deprived of attention and affection because of her mother's depression. She was an emotionally needy child who came to the attention of a child guidance clinic by age three as a result of head banging, hair pulling, and excessive demands for her mother's attention. As a young child she had viewed herself as a boy and acted the part, and at the onset of puberty she had begun refusing to wear dresses. There was family conflict about her dressing like a boy, and she had become isolated from her peers. She came to psychiatric treatment after having requested a sex change operation. She was adament about having been born the wrong sex and indicated that she daydreamed about herself in a male role.

TREATMENT METHOD: Treatment involved individual and milieu therapy in an inpatient setting over a two-year period. Individual therapy sessions took place three times each week. Highlights of the treatment process are as follows. The patient was initially guarded and distrustful. She gradually became more free in expressing herself, and at one point she noted that she especially enjoyed it when other patients acted out anger. During the course of treatment, she explored her feelings about her family. She had idealized her father, but she began to see him as aloof and uninvolved, someone she couldn't really count on. She began to recognize how he unfairly projected all the blame for his marital difficulties onto his wife, and her feelings toward her mother became more positive. She was especially pleased with her mother's ability to stand on her own when, during the course of treatment, the parents separated.

In her initial presentation the patient appeared as a boy and expressed a strong desire for a sex change operation. She was disappointed when she discovered that this would not make her a "perfectly normal boy," capable of fathering children. During the course of therapy, she vacillated between clear statements that she was a boy and ambivalence about sexual identity. She went from occasionally wearing female clothes out of social necessity to some experimentation with feminine dressing, to ultimately taking pleasure in dressing as a girl. Her relationships with staff also reflected changes in her gender position. At first she was aloof and withdrawn but then developed a crush on a female staff member. Later she expressed admiration for a male staff member who was not intimidated by her anger, and ultimately she developed a crush on him.

It is important to note that though her parents expressed disapproval at her cross-dressing prior to hospital admission, they only slowly acknowledged changes that she made in the direction of more feminine dressing, and they did not strongly reinforce them. There were indications that her mother was not pleased by her emerging attraction to boys.

TREATMENT RESULTS: The effects of treatment were that the patient ultimately came to see herself as a girl, to dress in female clothes, and to be attracted to males. At a two-and-a-half-year follow-up, she continued to be interested in boys, although she was not involved with anyone in particular.

COMMENTARY: Treatment was effective in terms of its basic objectives, though it was not clear at follow-up whether or not the patient would ultimately establish a heterosexual relationship. The cost of treatment was undoubtedly high, and it seems likely that greater efficiency could have been achieved by more targeting of specific behaviors for systematic reinforcement, at least in the later stages of treatment. Training the parents in reinforcement psychology might also have made treatment progress more rapidly. But only gradually did the patient come to find feminine identity at all attractive, and a too vigorous application of reinforcement psychology to specific feminine behaviors could easily have been counterproductive.

SOURCE: Davenport, C. W., and Harrison, S. I. "Gender Identity Change in a Female Adolescent Transsexual." *Archives of Sexual Behavior,* 1977, *6,* 327-340.

Gender Identity Change in a Male

AUTHORS: D. H. Barlow, E. J. Reynolds, and W. S. Agras

PRECIS: Systematic modification of gender specific behaviors in an adolescent male transsexual

INTRODUCTION: Gender identity is manifest through a complex set of sex role behaviors involving gross motor movements, manner of speaking, thoughts, fantasies, and patterns of sexual arousal. Barlow and his colleagues carefully analyzed each of these components, breaking them down into specific responses that could be taught to an individual with gender identity disturbance.

CASE HISTORY: The patient was a seventeen-year-old male who for as long as he could remember had viewed himself as female and who had begun cross-dressing before age five. As a young boy he had preferred girls as playmates and had been interested in activities like knitting, crocheting, and cooking. Anatomically and in chromosome studies he was a normal male, but in his sexual fantasies he imagined himself as a woman having intercourse with a man.

TREATMENT METHOD: Initial attempts at modifying fantasies and patterns of sexual arousal were unsuccessful, and it was decided that treatment would have to begin with changes in effeminate mannerisms in sitting, standing, and walking. Appropriate behaviors were modeled by a male therapist and practiced by the patient with feedback from the therapist. To enhance feedback, the final practice in each therapy session was videotaped for playback at the beginning of the next session. Masculine patterns of sitting, walking, and standing were each taught separately, and the client had to master one before moving on to the next.

Characteristics of speech were also modified. Pitch and voice inflections were the targets. The client was taught to regulate pitch through muscle control, and he was encouraged to abandon his precise, clipped manner of speaking in favor of a more relaxed, slightly slurred speech pattern. During this part of treatment, self-statements like "I like being a boy" and "Good looking women turn me on" were used in speech practice. Patient and therapist reviewed audiotapes of therapy sessions together.

Social skills training was also employed in this phase of treatment. There was role playing and practice of appropriate behaviors for various social situations, such as between-class breaks at school. The goals were to increase eye contact, initiative in conversation, and appropriateness and duration of responses. Video playback was available following each practice. After discussion, the therapist reenacted the scene and it was again played back and discussed. The session ended with a final repeat of this exercise by the patient.

By the point in treatment when overt behavior was mostly masculine, thoughts and fantasies continued to be feminine. Fantasy training involved presentation of pictures of *Playboy* models with encouragement to fantasize sexual involvement with the young woman in the picture. The client was reinforced for maintaining fantasy for a set period of time, the criterion duration being increased each day. The client was also encouraged to fantasize about girls he met each day and to specify what attributes he found attractive. After heterosexual fantasy was established, heterosexual arousal became the target of treatment. Arousal responses to pictures of nude women were increased by following their presentation with pictures of nude men, which elicited a strong sexual response. Once female pictures became associated with arousal, sexual response to looking at male pictures was decreased by contingent shock and by exercises in imagining unpleasant consequences for homosexual arousal.

TREATMENT RESULTS: Elimination of feminine mannerisms led to increased comfort in interpersonal relationships. Following voice training, the patient began to express pleasure with his masculine behavior; and, subsequent to fantasy training, the desire to be a female sharply declined. Spontaneous heterosexual fantasies began to appear, and with changes in arousal pattern, mannerisms became even more masculine. Follow-up appointments were scheduled over the first year after completion of treatment. At six months, the pattern of heterosexual arousal persisted, and homosexual arousal was at a low level. At one year, there was no further gender identity confusion, masculine behaviors continued at a high level, and heterosexual arousal continued to predominate. The patient had a girlfriend with whom he engaged in light petting, and there was a high level of heterosexual fantasy.

COMMENTARY: The client initially showed no motivation to change gender identity and, in fact, had requested a sex change operation. Changes in mannerisms undertaken to reduce social conflict led to increased motivation for more far-reaching changes. Treatment was conducted on an outpatient basis, which was considerably less expensive than inpatient treatment would have been. The willingness of this young man to cooperate with treatment is unusual in cases of gender identity disturbance and was no doubt an important factor in the success reported.

SOURCE: Barlow, D. H., Reynolds, E. J., and Agras, W. S. "Gender Identity Change in a Transsexual." *Archives of General Psychiatry,* 1973, *28,* 569-576.

Transsexual Wishes for
Sex Reassignment Surgery

AUTHOR: L. M. Lothstein

PRECIS: Management of patients seeking sex reassignment surgery

INTRODUCTION: Because of its profound social and psychological impact and because some aspects are irreversible, a great deal of caution is necessary in evaluating requests for sex reassignment surgery. Lothstein describes personality attributes of a group of patients making this request and provides information concerning factors that directly or indirectly precipitate it. She offers suggestions regarding management for these patients.

Individuals with transsexual wishes have a strong desire to dress as and pass for members of the opposite sex. Many of the patients Lothstein studied reported an aggravation of this impulse in connection with personal loss, such as the death of a parent. Some commented on the calming effect of cross-dressing, and a few indicated a belief that cross-dressing could magically reunite them with a lost love object. Others revealed that adolescent sexual changes had led to severely aggravated distress about their anatomical sex or that adolescent masturbation had exacerbated dissatisfaction. For some who experienced homosexual attractions, the conviction that they were really members of the opposite sex alleviated feelings of anxiety about homosexuality.

The following considerations are emphasized as important in diagnosing transsexualism:

1. The diagnosis cannot properly be made until late in the adolescent period.

2. It is necessary that there be a clear desire to be a member of the opposite sex rather than delusional thinking about sexual identity, including a desire to have the genitals of the opposite sex.

3. This desire is frequently manifest in both daydreams and night dreams in which the individual is cast as a member of the opposite sex.

4. Transsexuals are frequently asexual in orientation, not being comfortable with either heterosexual or homosexual objects.

CASE HISTORY: Twenty-seven adolescents requesting sex reassignment surgery were evaluated. A number of these dropped out after the initial intake meeting, but more than half received complete intake evaluations consisting of psychological testing and extensive clinical interviews. All twenty-seven presented in acute crisis, showing such symptoms as depression, impulsivity, poor judgment, and low frustration tolerance. Some showed evidence of delusional thinking, and more than 25 percent were suicidal and required hospitalization.

TREATMENT METHOD: Identification of the life stresses that have led to the wish for sex reassignment surgery often diminishes the desire, giving the therapist time to focus on underlying conflicts. Thorough evaluation of the relationship between such conflicts and the desire for surgery is essential. For some, the best treatment is one that assists them in conflict resolution rather than in achieving anatomical change.

TREATMENT RESULTS: Of the twenty-seven patients evaluated, only two females and one male underwent surgery (two other females were still being considered). Surgical candidates were seen for an average of five years of evaluation and psychotherapy before surgery. Post-surgical adjustment was seen as satisfactory. There was no evidence of personality deterioration, emergence of psychotic thinking, or suicidal ideation at one-year follow-up.

COMMENTARY: Because of the irreversibility of some aspects of sex reassignment treatment as well as the obvious psychopathology of many individuals seeking such treatment, extensive assessment and psychotherapy over a period of years is a necessary prelude to surgery. Lothstein does a service in highlighting issues that should be the focus of diagnostic and treatment interventions.

SOURCE: Lothstein, L. M. "The Adolescent Gender Dysphoric Patient: An Approach to Treatment and Management." *Journal of Pediatric Psychology,* 1980, *5,* 93-109.

Additional Readings

Barlow, D. H., Abel, G. G., and Blanchard, E. B. "Gender Identity Change in Transsexuals." *Archives of General Psychiatry,* 1979, *36,* 1001-1007.

The authors provide follow-up data on a previously reported successful gender identity change in a seventeen-year-old transsexual male (see above digest of Barlow, Reynolds, and Agras, 1973). Follow-up carried out over a six-and-a-half-year period revealed stable adjustment. Motor behavior was predominantly masculine and masturbation fantasies were heterosexual. The patient was involved in a stable heterosexual relationship and anticipating marriage.

Two additional cases are also reported, both adult males living as women and receiving hormonal treatment as a prelude to sex change surgery. Both became fearful about being able to pass as women after surgery and decided on a course of gender identity therapy. Treatment was successful in one case but only partially successful in the other.

Newman, L. E. "Transsexualism in Adolescence: Problems in Evaluation and Treatment." *Archives of General Psychiatry*, 1970, *23*, 112-121.

Newman points out that adolescence is particularly a time of crisis for the transsexual because of the difficulty of reconciling self-perception with others' expectations and that, for some transsexuals, a sex change operation offers the best hope for successful identity formation. He presents the case of a young male transsexual who, with the onset of adolescent changes, realized it was almost too late for him to begin living the life of a girl. He started cross-dressing and dating, with the intention of killing himself when it was no longer possible to pass as a girl. He came to Newman's attention after a serious suicide attempt. Careful evaluation within the context of a psychotherapeutic relationship confirmed the diagnosis of transsexualism. Family acceptance was worked through in a series of family therapy sessions. With the acceptance and support of his family, the boy began experimenting with living as a girl, and arrangements were made for her to live with a relative and attend a new school. Subsequent estrogen treatment stimulated breast development and enhanced her confidence about her feminine role. Several years of psychiatric follow-up revealed a positive adjustment, and ultimately the family helped arrange for sex reassignment surgery.

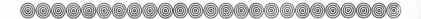

Homosexuality

Homosexual orientation develops throughout the childhood and adolescent years but may not come to awareness until adolescence or even later. Some individuals become quite distressed by homosexual impulses and seek treatment to change sexual orientation. Past sexual history and motivations and goals in seeking treatment must be carefully explored before treatment intervention. Treatment planning should include consideration of the need for change in arousal pattern, fantasy, and behavior. Interventions that have been effective include relaxation and desensitization, classical conditioning, positive reinforcement, and aversive training. A combination of approaches based on careful individualized assessment is most likely to be effective.

Self-Control Plus Aversive
Conditioning

AUTHOR: A. Canton-Dutari

PRECIS: A combination of self-control and aversive procedures used to decrease homosexual arousal and increase responsiveness to heterosexual stimuli

INTRODUCTION: Many individuals with a homosexual orientation are quite happy with this and have no desire for psychological treatment. Others experience conflict or dissatisfaction and some seek treatment to change sexual orientation. Treatment that emphasizes the teaching of self-control procedures to regulate sexual arousal reduces the danger that the therapist will attempt to impose his or her values and beliefs on these clients or to exercise control over their sexual behavior.

CASE HISTORY: Clients were fifty-four males aged thirteen to twenty-five who sought treatment for anxiety resulting from dissatisfaction with homosexual activity. They all regarded themselves as homosexuals and indicated that homosexual behavior had begun long before puberty. For these men, orgasm in the presence of another male occurred on an average of four times each week.

TREATMENT METHOD: Treatment involved a combination of several methods. The first session was devoted to instruction and practice in relaxation. Relaxation was accomplished through alternately tensing and releasing tension in various muscles and muscle groups. In the second session clients were taught how to inhibit orgasm when sexually aroused. This involved a three-step procedure: (1) contracting thighs strongly, (2) inhaling deeply, and (3) exhaling slowly while relaxing thighs.

During the initial three weeks of treatment, clients were instructed to use masturbation as their only sexual outlet and to use the "contraction-breathing method" to gain control over the length of time before orgasm. They were also asked to develop a hierarchy of sexually stimulating images based on past homosexual experiences. During the next several weeks, each client received aversive training for sexual arousal in the presence of homosexual stimuli (images from the hierarchy, photographs, and films). They were asked to signal sexual arousal whenever it occurred in the presence of these stimuli and received a mild, intermittent electric shock to the thigh until they began using the contraction-breathing method to decrease arousal. Despite aversive training, there was typically a rise in homosexual desire at about the ninth week, which was accompanied by the occurrence of nocturnal emissions. At that point clients were told that they should masturbate once each week and that they should allow orgasm only in the presence of heterosexual stimuli. Gradually over the next few weeks, nocturnal emissions began to occur in connection with heterosexual dream content.

In the final phase of treatment, the therapist began to shift emphasis in the therapy sessions toward discussion of the therapist-client relationship as an analog for male to male social relationships.

TREATMENT RESULTS: The vast majority (91 percent) of these clients did learn to control arousal in the presence of homosexual stimuli, and a majority (78 percent) experienced sexual arousal in the presence of heterosexual stimuli. Eleven remained exclusively heterosexual during a three-and-a-half-year follow-up period and eleven others did not revert to active homosexuality.

COMMENTARY: Canton-Dutari has demonstrated an effective method for control of sexual arousal and for influencing the nature of the stimuli that will elicit arousal. Although this method did help a number of men eliminate homosexual behavior and increase heterosexual behavior, not all those who showed a change in arousal pattern showed a corresponding behavioral change. For those who did not, some form of social skills training would probably have been beneficial. The importance of individual components of the treatment plan is uncertain. From the standpoint of avoiding possible coercive control, it would be best if aversive treatment could be eliminated. If it is essential, then clients should be helped to explore its probable consequences carefully so that informed consent can be obtained.

SOURCE: Canton-Dutari, A. "Combined Intervention for Controlling Unwanted Homosexual Behavior." *Archives of Sexual Behavior*, 1974, *3*, 367-371.

Desensitization in the Treatment of Homosexuality

AUTHOR: F. W. Huff

PRECIS: Increasing heterosexual behavior by decreasing fear of members of the opposite sex

INTRODUCTION: Huff reasoned that if fear of members of the opposite sex is a factor in homosexual adjustment, then eliminating such fears should increase the likelihood of heterosexual behavior. His approach to treatment was systematically to reduce such fears.

CASE HISTORY: The client was a nineteen-year-old male homosexual who also complained of stage fright. He became convinced of the anxiety component in his homosexuality when complying with the therapist's request to imagine himself in bed with a nude woman precipitated a severe anxiety attack. His anxiety hierarchy included sixteen items, ranging from having a conversation with several girls through such items as kissing a girl on lips and ultimately to items involving sexual intercourse.

TREATMENT METHOD: The first step in treatment was to es-

tablish a hierarchy of anxiety-arousing situations involving intimacy with the opposite sex. The client was taught deep muscle
relaxation and then taught to relax while imagining scenes from
this hierarchy. Scenes that evoked little anxiety were imagined
first and only when the client could think about them without
distress did he move on to the next item in the hierarchy. It
took eighteen sessions to reach the point at which he could relax while imagining all items in the hierarchy.

TREATMENT RESULTS: As therapy progressed, homosexual
fantasies and behaviors decreased to nearly zero and heterosexual fantasies and behaviors increased to the pretreatment frequency for homosexual fantasies and behaviors. The change was
maintained through a six-month follow-up.

COMMENTARY: Relaxation training was an effective tool in
the treatment of this young man seeking a change in sexual orientation. The authors do not distinguish between changes in
fantasy and changes in behavior in their data analysis; so the extent to which his behavior changed is unclear. However, it is
likely that for at least some clients, social skills training would
have to accompany desensitization to produce significant behavioral change.

SOURCE: Huff, F. W. "The Desensitization of a Homosexual."
Behavior Research and Therapy, 1970, *8,* 99-102.

Anticipatory Avoidance Learning

AUTHOR: D. E. Larson

PRECIS: Increasing heterosexual fantasies and behavior by pairing anticipatory homosexual behaviors with aversive consequences

INTRODUCTION: The use of aversive procedures in the treatment of homosexual impulses and behaviors often involves elaborate laboratory equipment. Larson describes the use of simple equipment that can be used in an office practice. The central idea of the therapy is to increase the relative power of heterosexual impulses by teaching the client to avoid anticipatory looking at or thinking about same sex partners.

CASE HISTORY: The client was an eighteen-year-old single male who had had thirty to forty homosexual experiences since his first experience at age fourteen. His interests and fantasies were homosexual, and he had never had heterosexual intercourse. He had stopped masturbating because the accompanying homosexual fantasies frightened him. Prior to treatment, he discussed with the therapist his feelings about homosexuality and his desire to move from homosexual to heterosexual behavior. He was warned that treatment would involve electric shock and told that there were no guarantees of success.

TREATMENT METHOD: Treatment involves the use of a 35-mm projector to display slides of potentially attractive males and females and a simple apparatus for delivering a shock to the tibial muscles of the leg. The client arranges the slides into a hierarchy of attractiveness, and the picture of the least attractive male is projected onto a screen, where it can be looked at or removed using a remote control switch. If the client does not remove it after eight seconds, he gets a shock, which is terminated as soon as he removes the slide. Each time a male picture is removed, a female picture is projected; so averting one's gaze from males and focusing on females becomes associated with relief of unpleasant shock. As treatment goes on, the attractiveness of the projected male pictures is increased. Female pictures are presented in reverse order. There were two sessions per week for five weeks. Each pair of male and female slides was presented twenty-five times and there were two different pairs presented in each session.

TREATMENT RESULTS: At the termination of treatment, the

client reported that he had heterosexual masturbation fantasies and also that his habit of looking at the genital region of other males had been eliminated. He had begun dating and enjoying physical intimacy with women. Four months after treatment, heterosexual impulses and fantasies continued, and he reported having had heterosexual intercourse several times with one woman. Monthly follow-up for one year was planned.

COMMENTARY: Homosexual impulses may become salient primarily because of a learned avoidance of the opposite sex. When a stronger avoidance reaction toward members of the same sex is promoted, sexual energies are then rechanneled into heterosexuality. If the original aversion is not too strong and if new behaviors are forthcoming and have a positive outcome, new habits are learned. However, in some cases, reduction of heterosexual anxiety may be necessary in addition. Also, social skills deficits may be so great that changes in sexual urges cannot be translated into new behaviors. Here again, specific therapies may have to be introduced. The clinician must be alert to these changing treatment needs and target his or her interventions accordingly.

With teenage clients especially, the therapist must consider values issues. The treatment goal is not necessarily that the client have heterosexual intercourse. Behavioral goals should be carefully explored with the client within the context of his or her own value system.

SOURCE: Larson, D. E. "An Adaptation of the Feldman and MacCulloch Approach to Treatment of Homosexuality by the Application of Anticipatory Avoidance Learning." *Behavior Research and Therapy*, 1970, *8*, 209-210.

A Social Learning Approach to the Treatment of Sexual Problems

AUTHOR: P. M. Bentler

PRECIS: Changing sexual orientation through behavioral rehearsal and changes in social and sexual consequences

INTRODUCTION: Traditional psychotherapies have brought little success in the treatment of homosexuality and transvestism. The author theorizes that this is because these learned behaviors are maintained by pleasurable consequences and also because corresponding fantasies that have become cues for sexual arousal are maintained by the pleasurable experience of orgasm during masturbation.

CASE HISTORY: Six case studies are reported, three involving homosexuals and three involving transvestites. Only two of the homosexual boys completed treatment. The first was a fourteen-year-old who had extensive homosexual fantasies but had had only one homosexual encounter. The second was a sixteen-year-old boy from a juvenile detention center who had a four-year history of homosexual fantasies and behavior and no heterosexual experience. None of the transvestite boys had either homosexual fantasies or experience. The youngest, age eleven, displayed markedly effeminate mannerisms, which became a major focus in his treatment. The therapist engaged him in playing ball and building model cars. During these activities, he systematically reinforced masculine behaviors and expressions while disapproving of effeminate mannerisms. The thirteen- and sixteen-year-old boys both used rolling on a bed in feminine clothing as a masturbation substitute.

In addition to the treatment to be described, they were given specific education regarding masturbation in an effort to decrease inhibition.

TREATMENT METHOD: Bentler's treatment plan has two phases. The first involves therapist-patient interviews focused on heterosexual behaviors. The therapist reinforces through attention and praise any patient verbalizations regarding interest in the opposite sex. Planning for heterosexual involvements is encouraged and appropriate social behaviors are rehearsed in the therapy session. Spontaneous expressions of heterosexual attraction as well as descriptions of social and sexual encounters are strongly reinforced. In the second phase of treatment, heterosexual behaviors that have been planned and rehearsed in therapy are carried out. These might include such things as focusing attention on that which is sexually attractive about a member of the opposite sex, engaging in heterosexual social interactions, dating, and expressing affection through physical intimacy. These activities provide material for fantasy, which is reinforced during subsequent masturbation.

TREATMENT RESULTS: For both homosexual boys who received treatment, homosexual fantasies decreased or were eliminated, and heterosexual behaviors increased. For the two older transvestite boys, cross-dressing ceased, masturbation with heterosexual fantasy increased, and social and sexual relationships with girls increased to "normal" levels. The youngest transvestite boy, who received a somewhat different treatment, showed an increase in masculine interests and friendships, decreased effeminate behavior, and elimination of cross-dressing.

COMMENTARY: This appears to be a direct and effective method for influencing sexual orientation. There are only minimal aversive consequences employed and the approach makes sense theoretically. Those planning to treat any of the problems described would do well to take a careful history regarding formal and informal experiences with sex education as well as a history of previous sexual behaviors and their consequences. With this information available, the therapist can plan for the alleviation of specific anxieties and inhibitions that may interfere with desired behaviors.

SOURCE: Bentler, P. M. "A Note on the Treatment of Adolescent Sex Problems." *Journal of Child Psychology and Psychiatry*, 1968, *9*, 125-129.

Aversion Therapy

AUTHORS: E. J. Callahan and H. Leitenberg

PRECIS: The influence of contingent shock and covert sensitization on sexual arousal, fantasy, and behavior

INTRODUCTION: Aversion therapies involve pairing an unpleasant event with the occurrence of a behavior that is to be decreased. Currently, the two most popular methods involve either low voltage electric shocks or directed imagination of unpleasant events (covert sensitization). When shock is used, it is generally administered as a punishment for undesirable behaviors or fantasies so that these will be suppressed or avoided. In covert sensitization the client is directed to imagine unpleasant events occurring simultaneously with or as a consequence of an undesirable behavior so that contemplating the behavior becomes unpleasant. Both these methods have been used to reduce or eliminate unwanted sexual impulses and behaviors. The authors of this article found covert sensitization to be the preferred approach.

CASE HISTORY: Several cases are presented; one was a nineteen-year-old homosexual male. He had a six-year history of homosexual behavior, and he sought treatment on the advice of friends and relatives. Initial treatment with shock failed to decrease homosexual urges or masturbation fantasies.

TREATMENT METHOD: All clients freely volunteered for treatment knowing that aversive methods would be used. They received both contingent shock and covert sensitization treatments. Initial covert sensitization sessions involved relaxation training so that scenes to be imagined could be presented while the client was in a relaxed state. Clients were interviewed to obtain specific information concerning sexually arousing imagery as well as related events they would consider particularly unpleasant; and in subsequent covert sensitization sessions, they were directed to imagine themselves engaged in the unwanted sexual behavior leading to an unpleasant consequence. Some

examples include finding syphilitic sores on a homosexual partner or being discovered by a friend or relative while engaged in
homosexual behavior. Each session involved the presentation of
four such scenes. In addition there were two scenes in which an
unpleasant consequence was avoided by terminating unwanted
behavior and approaching a heterosexual object.

TREATMENT RESULTS: For the nineteen-year-old male described above, using covert sensitization led to a decrease in
homosexual urges and fantasies and, after a three-month interruption in treatment, to increased heterosexual fantasy and behavior. These results were maintained through an eight-month
follow-up, at which point the client reported enjoyment in dating and petting with girls.

COMMENTARY: The treatment described was noticeably effective. It involved a number of components, each of which may
have contributed to the ultimate outcome, even though covert
sensitization produced the major effect. The support of family
and friends may well have been an important factor in success;
and one cannot discount the fact that all clients were preselected
for willingness to undergo aversive therapy; so motivation to
change was probably strong. This degree of commitment is important not only because it improves chances for success, but for
ethical reasons as well. With any client seeking changes in sexual
orientation or behavior, if one does not carefully establish motivation before embarking on a course of treatment, there is a danger of the therapist forgetting who the client is and becoming
the agent of the family or other cultural institution.
    Another important factor to be considered is the pace of
change. This young man apparently terminated treatment because changes were occurring more rapidly than he could assim-
ilate them. After a three-month hiatus, he was able to return
and successfully complete the treatment.

SOURCE: Callahan, E. J., and Leitenberg, H. "Aversion Ther-
    apy for Sexual Deviation: Contingent Shock and Covert Sen-

sitization." *Journal of Abnormal Psychology*, 1973, *81*, 60-73.

Additional Readings

Daher, D. "Sexual Identity Confusion in Late Adolescence: Therapy and Values." *Psychotherapy: Theory, Research and Practice*, 1977, *14*, 12-17.

    Daher describes an approach to therapy with late adolescents experiencing sexual identity confusion. His approach is based on the premise that most people are not exclusively homosexual or heterosexual, and he argues that the adolescent who is confused about his or her own preferences ought to explore feelings and fantasies freely and chose the orientation that suits him or her best. He allows clients to proceed at their own pace in bringing up sexual concerns, but once a concern has been expressed, he encourages clients to communicate explicitly about urges, fantasies, and behaviors. Once easy communication about the present has been established, details of sexual history are also explored. Clients are encouraged actively to pursue self-exploration outside the therapy hour through writing down experiences, experimenting with less inhibited manners of dressing, and engaging in visual self-exploration while naked. The emphasis is on clients becoming less constricted and developing a sense of freedom to consider what really is their preference. Daher cautions that the therapist who does not know or cannot accept his or her own sexual desires is in danger of manipulating the therapy to meet personal needs or of defensively seeking emotional distance from the client.

Gold, S., and Neufeld, I. L. "A Learning Approach to the Treatment of Homosexuality." *Behavior Research and Therapy*, 1965, *2*, 201-204.

    Gold and Neufeld report on the treatment of a sixteen-year-old male in trouble with the law for homosexual soliciting. Feelings of inadequacy were seen as central to his homosexual behavior. Treatment consisted of several components. First he was taught to relax while imagining himself in situations in which he feared failure. Later he was taught to imagine himself in situations in which he might solicit. The potential partner was described in an unattractive way, and the client was reinforced for indicating he would not solicit this person. Gradually, the partner was described in more attractive terms, but inhibiting factors, like the presence of a policeman, were introduced into the imagery. Finally, he was presented with choices between attractive males and females and reinforced for making "correct" choices. Cues that the choice of the male might lead to punishment were presented initially, but gradually faded out. Treatment was followed by elimination of the compulsion to make heterosexual contacts, increased success socially, and the beginnings of heterosexual dating.

◎◎◎◎◎◎◎◎◎◎◎◎◎◎◎◎◎◎◎◎◎◎◎◎◎◎

Exhibitionism and Voyeurism

*Both exhibitionism and voyeurism are classified as paraphilias,
disorders in which "unusual or bizarre imagery or acts are necessary for sexual excitement" (American Psychiatric Association,*
Diagnostic and Statistical Manual, *3rd ed., Washington, D.C.:
American Psychiatric Association, 1980). Exhibitionism, which
is probably the more common of the two, occurs only in males
and involves exposing the genitals to an unsuspecting female.
In voyeurism, sexual excitement is achieved by looking at unsuspecting people who are undressed or undressing or who are
engaged in sexual activity. In both disorders, the behavior necessary for sexual excitement is apt to bring the individual into
conflict with the law; so rapid behavior change is of paramount
importance. The person who engages in these activities frequently has inhibitions concerning more normal sexual behaviors or lacks the social skills to establish a relationship with an
appropriate partner.*

◎◎◎◎◎◎◎◎◎◎◎◎◎◎◎◎◎◎◎◎◎◎◎◎◎◎

Reinforcing an Alternative
to Exhibitionism

AUTHOR: L. F. Lowenstein

PRECIS: Eliminating exhibitionism by promoting an alternative mode of sexual expression

INTRODUCTION: Psychoanalytic theorists have viewed exhibitionism as a defensive behavior used to ward off unconscious castration fears. Lowenstein rejects this emphasis on unconscious motivations, preferring to focus on the maladaptive symptom behavior rather than on its possible causes and to work toward its elimination by promoting a competing behavior.

CASE HISTORY: The client was a seventeen-year-old unmarried male, referred by his probation officer. He was about to go to court in consequence of having exposed himself to some young girls. He had a long history of exhibitionism and engaged in this behavior several times a week. The urge was especially strong when he approached a wooded area and saw young girls playing. He indicated that he rarely masturbated, and he expressed an aversion to this "dirty" behavior.

TREATMENT METHOD: The first week of treatment was devoted to data collection. The client was asked to keep a daily diary, with particular emphasis on sexual stimulation and urges. At the end of one week, he was given instructions to masturbate daily while focusing on heterosexual fantasies. At the same time he was encouraged to keep busy and to spend as much time as possible with other people.

TREATMENT RESULTS: The result after twenty days was a decreased impulse toward exhibitionism and elimination of this behavior. This was maintained through a one-year follow-up, at which point the young man indicated that he felt quite certain he would not expose himself again. He did, however, mention "an inferiority complex" about his past behavior and expressed concern about limited dating and the lack of a steady girlfriend.

COMMENTARY: The therapist in this case encouraged his client to substitute a normal form of sexual expression for one that was bringing him into conflict with societal norms and laws. The client's lack of experience with masturbation made the elimination of the problem behavior much simpler than it might otherwise have been. In cases where the client already masturbates to exhibitionist fantasies, the problem is much more difficult to treat. Orgasm is a powerful reinforcer that promotes habits that anticipate its occurrence.

Although the treatment strategy was effective in eliminating the deviant behavior, it appears not to have gone far enough. Normal behavior for a seventeen-year-old boy also includes dating. This boy either had inhibitions about relationships with girls or lacked the social skills to follow through on his expressed wish to become more involved with them. Information concerning such problems should be elicited as part of the history of sexual development so that strategies for overcoming them can be made part of the overall treatment plan.

SOURCE: Lowenstein, L. F. "A Case of Exhibitionism Treated by Counterconditioning." *Adolescence*, 1973, *8*, 213-218.

Aversion Therapy for Exhibitionist Behavior

AUTHORS: M. J. MacColloch, C. Williams, and C. J. Birtles

PRECIS: Aversive treatment of exhibitionist behavior as part of a total therapy program

INTRODUCTION: Deviant sexual behavior has many determinants. Attraction to inappropriate objects or behaviors may develop when desired objects are forbidden or inappropriate objects are too available, and attraction is strengthened by the experience of orgasm associated with a particular behavior or fantasy about it. Lack of social skill may at least in part be responsible for avoidance of age appropriate behavior. Successful treatment of deviant sexual behaviors is enhanced by attention to the variety of influences that all together account for its occurrence.

CASE HISTORY: MacColloch and his colleagues present the case of a twelve-year-old boy who was sexually attracted to older women and who could not control the impulse to exhibit his genitals to them. This behavior usually occurred when he was alone and bored. He fantasized about older women with large breasts and buttocks and well-shaped legs, and he imagined himself exposing his erect penis to them. He would then undress himself and hide behind a curtain until an attractive woman passed by. At this point he would step into view, achieving orgasm when the woman appeared startled or masturbating afterwards to an exhibitionist fantasy.

TREATMENT METHOD: An attempt was made in verbal psychotherapy to overcome inhibitions about age appropriate sexual behavior, that is, attraction to and association with girls of a similar age. After two months of psychotherapy, the boy was able to talk more freely about sexuality, but he was still unable to resist the impulse to expose himself to an older woman. After several more months of therapy, he reported that he had not been involved in any further exhibitionistic behavior, that his masturbation fantasies were no longer exhibitionistic, and that he was becoming increasingly interested in girls his own age. However, another incident two months later led to a decision that, in addition to encouraging age appropriate behavior, the therapist should work directly on decreasing the boy's impulses to expose himself.

Because fantasizing about older women appeared to be the stimulus for a chain of thoughts and behaviors leading up to exhibitionism, the goal of aversive treatment was to help the client to avoid such imagery. This was accomplished in the following way. First a series of eight pictures of attractive older women was prepared and rank ordered in terms of increasing attractiveness. Then a similar series of pictures of same-age girls was prepared and rank ordered in terms of decreasing attractiveness. The picture of the least attractive woman was presented on a slide projector the client could control by advancing to the picture of the most attractive girl his own age. If he failed to change pictures within eight seconds, he received a mild electric shock, but if he made the change, the habit of visualizing a girl his own age was strengthened by shock avoidance. After he had learned to switch the picture consistently, the consequences were modified slightly to strengthen the habit. On the basis of a random program built into the apparatus, attempts to activate the switch no longer worked immediately on every occasion, and sometimes they did not work at all, so that shock was received. This kind of intermittent success was designed to approximate the real-world conditions with which this client would ultimately be faced. These same procedures were applied using all pictures in the two series.

TREATMENT RESULTS: Altogether there were eighteen twenty-minute treatment sessions. At the end of treatment, the boy reported he was able to control the start of the chain of thought that in the past had led to his exhibiting himself, but he indicated that he still had some exhibitionist masturbatory fantasy. At six-week follow-up these fantasies had been eliminated and compulsive thoughts about exhibiting himself were also absent. At five-month follow-up this was still the case, and he reported that he had a girlfriend and was less anxious about heterosexual relationships.

COMMENTARY: Aversive treatment occurred within the context of an already existing therapy relationship. The cumulative effect of treatment was that the client was able to avoid exhibiting himself and begin engaging in the age appropriate behavior that had been the focus of the beginning phase of treatment. Treatment started this client on a desired couse, and he was able to continue to make progress even after treatment sessions were discontinued.

SOURCE: MacColloch, M. J.,Williams, C., and Birtles, C. J. "The Successful Application of Aversion Therapy to an Adolescent

Exhibitionist." *Journal of Behavior Therapy and Experimental Psychiatry,* 1971, 2, 61-66.

Additional Readings

Jackson, B. T. "A Case of Voyeurism Treated by Counter Conditioning." *Behavior Research and Therapy,* 1969, 7, 133-134.

Jackson reviews the case of a twenty-year-old male who had been peeping in windows for about five years with the objective of observing nude females. The client was helped to substitute looking at nude pictures for peeping in windows. He was advised that when he felt the urge to peep, he should retire to his bedroom and look at a pornographic picture he found very exciting sexually and to accompany this looking with masturbation. After two weeks, he reported no further urge to look in windows, and at that point he was advised to substitute *Playboy* pictures for the pornographic picture. There were no further impulses to look in windows during the remaining six weeks of treatment. Results of long-term follow-up are unclear, but the urge to look in windows was diminished, if not completely eliminated.

Rooth, F. G., and Marks, I. M. "Persistent Exhibitionism: Short-Term Response to Aversion, Self Regulation and Relaxation Treatments." *Archives of Sexual Behavior,* 1974, 4, 227-248.

Rooth and Marks report on a study comparing various methods of treatment for exhibitionism. Patients were twelve males ranging in age from eighteen to fifty-three. All reported difficulties in their heterosexual relationships, such as impotence and premature ejaculation. Vocationally, they were underachievers, and many had problems, such as violent temper outbursts, in social relationships. The most effective of the three treatments studied was aversion therapy, involving shocks to the patient's forearm while he imagined himself exposing or during actual rehearsals of exposure. Cure was not complete in that seven patients did engage in some exhibitionism during a six-month follow-up period, but the rate of exposing was significantly less after treatment, and attitudes toward exposing were less positive.

Sexual Trauma

For the victim of rape, there is lasting emotional impact that may drastically influence subsequent development. Effects include specific anxieties and defensive behaviors as well as lowered self-esteem and feelings of worthlessness. Similar effects may occur for the victim of incest. Appropriate intervention can mitigate the impact of such trauma and decrease its long-term effects, but anxiety and overreaction on the part of those charged with helping the victim can and often do aggravate the problem. Especially in the case of parental incest, excessive zeal in protecting the child from the offending parent may lead to inappropriate separation and placement, leaving the child with the feeling that he or she is being punished for taking part in the incestuous relationship.

Specific Therapies for the Victim
of Sexual Trauma

AUTHOR: R. Wolff

PRECIS: Specific therapeutic interventions for overcoming emotional disturbance in the victim of a rape attempt

INTRODUCTION: The experiencing of unexpected traumatic events can lead to emotional and behavioral reactions that continue long after the precipitating events have occurred. The elimination of these anxiety reactions and defensive behaviors requires specifically targeted interventions.

CASE HISTORY: The client was a twenty-year-old woman who had been the victim of a rape attempt at age thirteen. Her story, given at the time of the event, was not initially believed; and by the time it was accepted, she was no longer willing to discuss the matter, even though a therapist was provided. The after-effects of the trauma were fear of the dark, fear of being alone, difficulty sleeping, and compulsive checking for an intruder whenever she entered an empty room. Checking involved thirteen separate steps, such as opening closets, looking under beds, and looking into the kitchen. The habits were quite strong even seven years after the precipitating incident.

TREATMENT METHOD: The first problem to be addressed was the sleep disturbance. The client was taught how to gain self-control of body tension through deliberate tensing and relaxing of various muscle groups. Once she had learned how to achieve a state of relaxation, she was directed to relax while imagining events progressively more like the original sexual trauma. As she mastered less frightening scenes, the more frightening ones were introduced.

To overcome her habit of compulsive checking for intruders, the therapist directed her to overuse this defensive behavior. Each time she entered an empty room, she was to carry out all checks, go outside and lock the door, and then return to do them all over again. She was instructed to repeat this five separate times. After doing it for one week, she was given the option of not checking at all or continuing to make all checks five times.

TREATMENT RESULTS: After four treatment sessions, her problems with insominia were greatly diminished. Compulsive checking was quickly eliminated under the free choice condition.

COMMENTARY: This case illustrates the relative permanence of anxiety reactions to sexual trauma and points out the need for specific interventions to deal with their various components. Without such intervention, this young woman would probably have continued indefinitely with habits that were a great nuisance to her and that seriously interfered with her freedom. The fact that the entire course of her adolescent years was influenced by this traumatic event points up the need for crisis intervention therapies for rape victims and also for follow-up once a crisis has passed. Greater sensitivity and compassion at the time of the attack would have helped this young girl work through her emotional reaction more easily and would probably have made it possible for her to experience a more normal adolescence.

SOURCE: Wolff, R. "Systematic Desensitization and Negative Practice to Alter the After Effects of a Rape Attempt." *Journal of Behavior Therapy and Experimental Psychiatry*, 1977, *8*, 423-425.

Special Issues in Therapy for Incest Victims

AUTHORS: M. J. Krieger, A. A. Rosenfeld, A. Gordon, and M. Bennett

PRECIS: Discusses possible pitfalls in psychotherapy with children who have been involved in incestuous relationships

INTRODUCTION: Krieger and her colleagues note that children who have been involved in incestuous relationships often present in their initial therapy contacts as flirtatious and seductive and as overly anxious to please the therapist. They illustrate with case material the common phenomena of "accidental" genital contact, exposure of underclothing, and suggestive remarks. Several possible explanations are offered for these behaviors:

1. The children's experience may lead them to expect that needs for attention or nurturance will be satisfied only through sexual encounters.
2. To ward off anxiety about being a passive victim, the child may take an active role in the seduction, which is felt to be inevitable.
3. The child may be testing the safety of the therapy situation before venturing to discuss sexual experiences.

SPECIAL CONSIDERATIONS IN TREATMENT: It is not unusual for therapists to be sexually stimulated by the behavior of these clients, however strong taboos against such feelings may lead to repression and denial. To bolster his or her own defenses, the therapist may become emotionally distant and fail to perceive the client's attempts to bring up sexual material. The therapist may also become overzealous in blaming the parent or parents and biased in clinical judgments regarding family involvement and issues of child placement. Other possible complications include being manipulated into granting special favors or failing to enforce normal limits.

The immediate goal for therapy is allow the client to express feelings and to experience acceptance. Not only feelings
regarding the incest experience are important, but also feelings
of fear or deprivation that may have prompted acquiescence in
the incestuous relationship. It is to be expected that as the client begins to deal with this material, angry feelings will also
emerge and may be displaced onto the therapist. In order to respond effectively, the therapist must remain open to and accepting of his or her own feelings. Responses must be consistent
and predictable so that the client learns the therapist is in control of his or her own impulses and will not be either seduced or
driven away.

COMMENTARY: Although Krieger and her colleagues do not
discuss specific therapy techniques, the issues they raise are vi-
tally important to the development of a therapeutic relationship. Once a relationship has been established, feelings can be
freely discussed and alternative ways of satisfying unmet needs
can be explored. In addition, the likelihood of discovering specific deficits in such areas as social skills or academic performance is quite high, and these may also become an important
focus in treatment. Other members of the family require their
own treatment, including marital therapy; and family sessions
are probably necessary to work through feelings and to clarify
and reinforce appropriate boundaries in family relationships.

SOURCE: Krieger, M. J., Rosenfeld, A. A., Gordon, A., and
    Bennett, M. "Problems in the Psychotherapy of Children
    with Histories of Incest." *American Journal of Psychother-
    apy*, 1980, *34*, 81-88.

Social Skills Training for a Sexually Aggressive Male

AUTHORS: S. M. Turner and V. B. Van Hasselt

PRECIS: Social skills training for a sexually aggressive male with problems in establishing normal social relationships

INTRODUCTION: Decreasing the incidence of sexual trauma requires appropriate treatment for sexually aggressive males. It has been noted that those who commit rape often show serious social skills deficits that prevent them from establishing normal social relationships with women. Turner and Van Hasselt describe a social skills training program for such an individual.

CASE HISTORY: The patient was a seventeen-year-old male who had followed an unknown woman to an isolated area of a park and attempted to rape her. She succeeded in getting away, and he was not apprehended. He later came for treatment because he was preoccupied with thoughts about the incident and because he was afraid he might do it again. In fact, he often engaged in "trailing" women, at times with the clear purpose of catching them alone.

TREATMENT METHOD: Treatment involved two components, self-monitoring and social skills training. Self-monitoring quickly eliminated obsessive thoughts, and the focus shifted to social skills training, with an emphasis on deficiencies noted during behavioral assessment. Target behaviors included eye contact, rate of speech, speech intonation, smiling, use of positive statements, and appropriateness of affect and speech content. Treatment for deficiencies in these areas was begun sequentially rather than all at once and involved modeling, behavioral rehearsal, direct instruction, feedback, and verbal reinforcement.

Rehearsal was carried out through simulated social interactions with a female confederate of the therapist. The patient and the young woman were seated in a room together, and the scene was set by narration over an intercom connected with an adjoining room. For example, the patient was asked to imagine himself in a school cafeteria looking for a seat and finding a girl seated at an otherwise unoccupied table. He was asked to make an opening remark, to which the confederate responded in a prearranged fashion, obligating him to respond again. There were ten scenes, five in which the patient took the initiative and five in which the confederate made the first move. There were sixteen half-hour treatment sessions over a period of eight weeks. Subsequently, there was a course of inpatient treatment for compulsive hand washing and other ritualistic behaviors.

TREATMENT RESULTS: As noted previously, obsessive thoughts were quickly eliminated. There were also changes in social skills manifest in increased eye contact, smiling, and use of positive statements. At eight-month follow-up, the patient reported less anxiety and greater self-confidence in relationships with women, and he had had several dates since termination of treatment. He had made no further attempts at sexual assault and was not seriously bothered by thoughts about doing so.

COMMENTARY: This article illustrates the important treatment strategy of decreasing problem behaviors by strengthening deficit behaviors. Although in this case such an approach did lead to a decrease in sexual aggression, other sources of aggressive impulse might also have to be explored in some cases, with the patient being helped to channel anger into constructive problem solutions.

SOURCE: Turner, S. M., and Van Hasselt, V. B. "Multiple Behavioral Treatment in a Sexually Aggressive Male." *Journal of Behavior Therapy and Experimental Psychiatry,* 1979, *10,* 343-348.

Additional Readings

Anant, S. "Verbal Aversion Therapy with a Promiscuous Girl: A Case Report." *Psychological Reports,* 1968, *22,* 795-796.

Anant presents the case of a twenty-year-old retarded woman who was unable to hold a job because of sexual promiscuity. She readily took up with anyone who showed the least interest in her, often leaving right in the middle of the work day. She was felt to be at risk for sexual abuse, venereal disease, and pregnancy. Treatment involved imagining anxiety-arousing scenes of worst possible outcomes, like being murdered by a sex criminal or contracting syphilis. The girl was also taught relaxation skills so that once a high level of anxiety was attained in imagining these outcomes, she could voluntarily return to a state of relaxation. There were ten treatment sessions, after which the patient took a new job, which she still retained at eight-month follow-up.

James, K. L. "Incest: The Teenager's Perspective." *Psychotherapy: Theory, Research and Practice,* 1977, *14,* 146-155.

This article describes treatment for seven teenage girls who had earlier experienced an incestuous relationship with a father or stepfather. One was treated individually and the other six met in groups of three. There were eight one-hour sessions with topics for discussion chosen at a beginning planning meeting. Topics included feelings toward the parent involved, understanding of his motivations, feelings toward males in general, feelings about rape, reactions to talking about the incident, self-image, and personal sensitivities. No statistical analysis is presented, but results suggest that as a result of group discussion, girls felt more comfortable in talking about their experience and more positive about themselves. They all indicated that the services offered to them immediately after they revealed the incest had been inappropriate and harmful and that what would have been most helpful was family counseling sessions.

@@

Teenage Pregnancy

Unwanted pregnancy in the adolescent years is a major social problem. For the mother-to-be, it may lead to the physical and psychological risks of an abortion or to limitations in future development as a result of early assumption of parenthood. For the babies, there are increased risks of birth complications and congenital defects as well as the risk of a host of problems associated with inadequate parenting throughout their developmental years. Despite these risks, sexual intercourse between young teenagers is a frequent phenomenon, and the majority of sexual encounters probably do not involve protection against pregnancy. Easy access to birth control has not solved the problem. Successful interventions have emphasized improving interpersonal skills and within-family communication.

@@

308

Pregnancy Prevention

AUTHORS: L. D. Gilchrist, S. P. Schinke, and B. J. Blythe

PRECIS: A pregnancy prevention program involving group training in social skills

INTRODUCTION: Neither an understanding of the adverse consequences of pregnancy nor knowledge of birth control methods is any guarantee that sexually active teenagers will use effective contraception. Knowledge must be transformed into personal decisions, which in turn must be implemented through specific behaviors. Gilchrist and his colleagues have designed a three-part intervention package to prevent teenage pregnancy that takes into account all these elements.

TREATMENT METHOD: From a group of twenty-one female and fifteen male high school sophomores, half were picked at random to participate in the training program (the others served as controls for evaluation studies). Groups met twice weekly for seven weeks. Basic information was provided through a film on adolescent sexuality and through lectures, demonstrations, and discussions of human reproduction and birth control. There were homework assignments involving information gathering at local community agencies and periodic quizzes to ensure accurate learning.

Once basic information had been mastered, the goal was to make it personally relevant by exploring specific applications. One such application involved discussing contraception with a dating partner. Group members identified potential obstacles and generated plans for overcoming them. They talked about such things as handling embarrassment and dealing with the partner's reaction. Group leaders modeled good communication skills and gave instruction, feedback, and social reinforcement. Specific goals included learning to initiate discussion, disclose feelings, refuse unreasonable demands, and request changes in another's behavior.

In the final stage of training, participants practiced new

skills outside the treatment setting. Homework assignments were given as a prerequisite to successful completion of the program. These included such things as buying condoms or foam at a drug store, visiting a family planning counselor, or actually talking about contraception with a boyfriend or girlfriend.

TREATMENT RESULTS: Trainees scored higher on tests concerning human reproduction and contraception and on tests of interpersonal problem solving than did untrained peers. They also scored higher on a videotaped communication test, showing more eye contact, ability to say no to others, and ability to request others to change their behavior. At six-month follow-up, trainees showed more consistent use of contraceptives, fewer incidents of unprotected intercourse, and greater use of contraceptives at last intercourse.

COMMENTARY: The program outlined produced a clear impact in a brief time span. The authors also demonstrated application of their general prevention strategy to the problem of pre-adolescent smoking and suggested a variety of other problems likely to yield to such an approach, including delinquency, alcohol consumption, and eating disturbances.

SOURCE: Gilchrist, L. D., Schinke, S. P., and Blythe, B. J. "Primary Prevention Services for Children and Youth." *Children and Youth Services Review*, 1979, *1*, 379-391.

Factors Affecting Contraceptive Practices

AUTHORS: M. H. Dembo and B. Lundell

PRECIS: Discussion of factors affecting adolescent contraceptive practices and suggestions for improving sex education programs

INTRODUCTION: Despite the multitude of problems resulting from unwanted pregnancies, large numbers of sexually active teenagers never use contraception. Although some lack information about birth control, providing information has not solved the problem. Dembo and Lundell stress cognitive-emotional development and attitudes toward sexuality as important limiting factors affecting the teenager's utilization of available information.

Adolescence is a time of transition from concrete to formal operations thinking. The latter involves the ability to anticipate future consequences and to plan for them. For the teenager who has not yet achieved this level of cognitive maturity, immediate concerns like avoiding the self-censure involved in planning for a sexual encounter weigh much more heavily than avoidance of the negative consequence of a pregnancy, an event seen as only remotely possible. The egocentricity of adolescent thinking is also important. Many teenagers have difficulty with applying what they know in general to their own specific situation. They assume that they are somehow the exception and that although others might get pregnant, they probably will not.

Attitudes toward sexuality are still another factor. If sex is bad, it certainly should not be planned for. Sometimes it may happen by accident, but one is not personally responsible. Those individuals who believe in their personal right to make choices about sexual behavior are more likely to use contraceptive information. Those who are negative and anxious about sexuality will not.

TREATMENT METHOD: Dembo and Lundell discuss a number of strategies for improving the outcome of sex education programs:

1. Sex education programs should be more broadly educational, including discussion of community standards for behavior and responsible decision making.

2. There should be more emphasis on the adolescent's immediate personal concerns, including discussion of such topics as masturbation, orgasm, homosexuality, and pornography.

3. Peer discussion groups should be utilized as a means of breaking down egocentric thinking.

4. Educators should involve parents to a much greater degree.

5. Programs should be designed to accommodate individual differences with respect to cognitive-emotional development and attitudes toward sexuality.

COMMENTARY: Dembo and Lundell provide important insights as to why sexually active teenagers often fail to use birth control. They also discuss ways of remedying this problem. It is, however, possible that improved education may not be able to overcome all obstacles. Bolstering externally imposed standards of behavior is probably a necessary stop gap, until the teenager reaches a level of maturity at which he or she is capable of responsible decision making.

SOURCE: Dembo, M. H., and Lundell, B. "Factors Affecting Adolescent Contraceptive Practices: Implications for Sex Education." *Adolescence,* 1979, *14,* 657-664.

Contraceptive Risk Taking

AUTHORS: H. Harari, T. Harari, and K. Hosey

PRECIS: Explores reasons for failure to use contraceptives among sexually active teenagers

INTRODUCTION: Birth control information and contraceptive devices are accessible to most young women, but the incidence of unplanned and unwanted pregnancies continues to rise. Harari and his co-workers sought an explanation for this phenomenon by asking known contraceptive rejectors in mental health clinics and in a "normal" population "why don't you use contraceptives?"

RESEARCH FINDINGS: The answers fell clearly into three categories: "clinical-interpersonal," "political-economic," and "situational." The clinical-interpersonal category included such responses as "maybe the baby will love me, since everybody else rejects me" and "this is one way of getting back at my parents." The political-economic included responses like, "welfare will set me up and I'll be sitting pretty" and "contraceptives are just another way of reducing the number of minorities." Fears about contraceptive side effects were included under the situational category.

The first two categories accounted for most of the responses, regardless of whether the respondent came from a mental health clinic or from the normal sample, and there was almost no difference in response between these two groups. What did emerge was a difference between blacks and whites, with whites generally offering a clinical-interpersonal explanation and blacks generally offering a political-economic explanation. The authors suggest that the teenagers in their study are simply making the responses that society expects them to make on the bases of social sterotypes and that these stereotypes indeed influence their behavior.

COMMENTARY: The groups under study are somewhat specialized. These are girls who actively reject contraception. Not all teenagers know their own minds so decisively. Some get pressured into sexual relations they didn't intend to have and don't have time to take precautions. Some have little capacity for projecting themselves into the future and simply don't consider taking precautions. Also, for some teenagers, pregnancy may at least temporarily solve certain problems of adolescent development. Motherhood may be the only adult role available or may be the only route to resources for establishing independence.

SOURCE: Harari, H., Harari, T., and Hosey, K. "Contraceptive Risk-Taking in White and Black Unwed Females." *The Journal of Sex Research*, 1979, *15*, 56-63.

A Multimodal Approach to the Prevention
of Repeat Pregnancies

AUTHORS: P. N. Kaufman and A. L. Deutsch

PRECIS: Group therapy, parent counseling and education, and staff consultation as components of a total program for the prevention of repeat pregnancies

INTRODUCTION: The problems associated with teenage pregnancies are compounded when teenage mothers have a second child. Kaufman and Deutsch concluded that a program for preventing repeat pregnancies would have the greatest chance for success if it were integrated with prenatal care for the first pregnancy. The target group would be a captive audience, dependent upon hospital staff for physical care. Resistance to psychological intervention would be reduced if it were introduced under the mantle of a comprehensive health care program, and the total resources of that program could be utilized. Parents of the pregnant adolescent would be more available for intervention during the pregnancy than at any point afterwards.

CASE HISTORY: Group members were enrolled in a prenatal clinic at a large city hospital. Only unmarried girls between the ages of twelve and sixteen who were experiencing their first pregnancy were eligible for membership. From a pool of twenty, eight were selected at random. Seven of these had mothers who had also had out of wedlock pregnancies. All the girls were attending school, though in most cases attendance was sporadic and performance was poor.

TREATMENT METHOD: The core of the treatment program was a group meeting held on a weekly basis. The focus changed with changes in the participants' needs. The problem was initially one of establishing a relationship between therapist and clients and building group cohesiveness. The group subsequently became a forum for discussing frustrations and anxieties regarding pregnancy and delivery. The therapist facilitated group interaction, functioned as a communication channel to parents and other clinic staff, and was consistently available as an emotional support. Therapy continued for more than a year after delivery, focusing on such issues as dating, work, care of the baby, family planning, and family communication problems. Throughout therapy, individual mother-daughter sessions were scheduled as needed to resolve specific communication problems.

The therapist began her relationship with the girls by feeding them milkshakes and cookies during the early meetings. As they became more free to express themselves, they focused on their feelings that they were treated poorly by clinic staff because they were unmarried. The therapist used this as an opportunity to demonstrate that the system could be responsive to them. Meetings between the therapist and other clinic staff helped them to understand the girls better and changed their behavior toward them. The girls also complained about their mothers' attitudes toward them. Mothers apparently felt that keeping their distance emotionally and reacting punitively would discourage their daughters from repeating their mistakes. Groups meetings with mothers as well as individual mother-daughter sessions reduced communication problems and helped the mothers be more supportive. As staff and mothers changed their behavior toward the girls, the girls became more available to looking at their part in problem interactions.

TREATMENT RESULTS: At the end of a year and a half of treatment, the group was terminated. There had been no repeat pregnancies, as contrasted with nine in the untreated group of twelve girls. Four girls were working at jobs they had held for at least six months; one was in school; and the others were staying home and taking care of their babies.

COMMENTARY: This highly successful, easy to implement program should be widely imitated. Those implementing such a program would do well to pay careful attention to therapist selection, as the therapist's personality and interpersonal skills appear crucial to program success. The therapist's commitment to a long-term, continuous relationship is probably a very important factor in program success. Although social skills training is not emphasized in the description of this program, it seems likely that a good deal of it occurred both as part of the ongoing interaction between group members and when the group focused on problem interactions with family and clinic staff.

SOURCE: Kaufman, P. N., and Deutsch, A. L. "Group Therapy for Pregnant Unwed Adolescents in the Prenatal Clinic of a General Hospital." *International Journal of Group Psychotherapy*, 1967, *17*, 309-320.

The Evolution of a Therapeutic Group

AUTHOR: B. B. Braen

PRECIS: The evolution of a therapeutic group for pregnant school-age girls within the context of a comprehensive educational and medical program

INTRODUCTION: Braen reports on group therapy conducted as part of a comprehensive program for pregnant school-age girls. In addition to psychological services, this program included obstetric, pediatric, educational, social work, and nursing services. With several years experience, an approach to group therapy that effectively engaged students and promoted meaningful communication evolved. Braen shares the experiences and thinking leading to the changes that occurred.

CASE HISTORY: In order to enter the program a girl had to be pregnant, under 21 and not yet graduated from high school. Participants tended to be primarily girls from lower socioeconomic levels who were unmarried and pregnant for the first time. Girls ranged in age from 11 to 21, and median age declined from 18.5 to 16.5 over the three-year period that formed the basis for this report.

TREATMENT METHOD: In the first year, girls met in groups of eight on a weekly basis. The groups had been created to provide a forum for discussing such issues as parents' attitudes toward the pregnancy, foster care for the babies, and responsibilities of the babies' fathers. Group leaders' orientation was primarily passive and reflective. They were content to let the agenda develop spontaneously during the course of the therapy hour.

After several months, the therapists decided that this approach was not working. The girls needed more structure and direction, and they seemed to want the therapist to reveal himself or herself before risking their trust in the therapist. To solve these problems, a major modification was made in the format for group meetings. Group therapy was integrated with the educational program and small groups were abandoned in favor of a "psychology class." Each class began with a presentation by the therapist that served to focus discussion for the remainder of the hour. Classes covered such topics as "reasons for intercourse, reasons for pregnancy, contraception, rape, incest, mothering, fathering, surrender, adoption, divorce, love, and dreams." As the year progressed and relationships developed, therapists tended to present less and less formally, and, at least for while, group discussion increased.

A problem developed in the second half of the academic year. Many girls who came into the program during the year were participating without benefit of the more structured sessions that had gone before, and they failed to become interested or involved. The solution adopted was to adhere closely in all meetings to the successful format of brief lecture followed by discussion and to repeat in the second semester all those topics covered in the first.

COMMENTARY: With several years experience, an effective model was developed for engaging school-age pregnant girls in a therapeutic group. The familiar structure of "a class" provided a safe forum for therapists and students to get to know each other. Class topics were of such emotional significance that group discussion developed naturally. The relationships that developed with therapists in class also made them more accessible to class participants for individual therapy contacts outside of class. An interesting comment on the value of the approach is that eventually all the other disciplines (obstetrics, pediatrics, social work, and nursing) came to use a similar format for their presentations.

SOURCE: Braen, B. B. "The Evolution of a Therapeutic Group Approach to School-Age Pregnant Girls." *Adolescence,* 1970, *5,* 171-186.

Teenage Mothers Seeking Jobs

AUTHORS: S. P. Schinke, L. D. Gilchrist, T. E. Smith, and S. E. Wong

PRECIS: Behavioral training for teenage mothers to improve their ability to compete for jobs

INTRODUCTION: Pregnant teenagers who decide to keep their babies must often depend upon public assistance for their income. For most, improved socioeconomic standing will come only through paying jobs; but finding employment opportunities, successfully completing applications and interviews, and keeping the job obtained all present obstacles. Schinke and his colleagues have developed a program to help teenage mothers secure available jobs through successful applications and interviews.

All participants were mothers or mothers-to-be enrolled in a high school continuation program for pregnant teenagers. The majority were black, though a few were white or hispanic. Most were single.

TREATMENT METHOD: Training took place in four weekly ninety-minute sessions. Thorough pretesting was carried out to determine specific weakness in completing applications and participating in interviews. Behavior training was directed toward general issues as well as specific weaknesses of individual participants. Training sessions on completing applications emphasized issues like reading application forms carefully, clarifying unfamiliar terms or confusing instructions, and providing information in a neat and orderly fashion. Training for employment interviews emphasized such things as answering questions in a clear and concise manner, presenting past employment favorably, and highlighting strong points of academic background. Group leaders used instruction and demonstration to convey appropriate behaviors, and participants practiced in pairs playing out the roles of interviewer and interviewee. Group leaders observed interactions, providing evaluation and feedback, coaching, and verbally reinforcing successful performance. All training sessions were followed by refreshments.

TREATMENT RESULTS: Employment applications completed by those who had received behavioral training were neater than those of a comparable control group and demonstrated better academic preparation, more positive employment histories, and greater competence than those of the untrained. On videotapes of simulated interviews, those who had received behavioral training showed more eye contact, more positive self-statements, fewer negative self-statements, more neutral informative statements, and fewer inappropriate responses. Having reviewed application forms and videorecordings of simulated interviews, trained personnel counselors found them to be much more likely candidates for employment than their control peers.

COMMENTARY: Schinke and his colleagues had very clear objectives for this program. They were aware of specific behaviors that affect success in the job application process, and they conducted realistic pretests to identify specific weaknesses, which became the focus for training sessions. When the issue is skills deficits, this is the kind of approach most likely to succeed. Similar training programs need to be designed to teach skills necessary for finding employment opportunities and for holding a job once it has been obtained.

SOURCE: Schinke, S. P., Gilchrist, L. D., Smith, T. E., and Wong, S. E. "Improving Teenage Mother's Ability to Compete for Jobs." *Social Work Research and Abstracts*, 1978, *14*, 25-29.

Additional Readings

Finkel, M. L., and Finkel, D. J. "Male Adolescent Contraceptive Utilization." *Adolescence*, 1978, *13*, 443-451.

The authors explore contraceptive use among a large group of sexually active urban high school students. Sixty-nine percent of a total of 421 male students reported that they were sexually experienced. Only 15 percent of these always used condoms, though about 35 percent did so at least some of the time. White males showed more effective use of contraceptives in general and more frequent use of condoms in particular than did their black and hispanic peers. Age was an important variable in that two thirds of those fifteen and younger were ineffective contraceptors and two thirds of the eighteen- and nineteen-year-olds were effective. The most frequently given reason for not using condoms was not having one available, suggesting that intercourse was often unplanned. With nearly 25 percent of the sample, however, condom use was seen as just not important. The authors suggest the use of peer group rap sessions as a means of conveying knowledge about contraceptive methods and motivating their use.

Rosen, R. H. "Adolescent Pregnancy Decision Making: Are Parents Important?" *Adolescence*, 1980, *15*, 43-54.

Rosen provides data concerning the extent to which teen-agers involve their parents in decisions concerning unwanted pregnancies. Despite the fact that most of the girls studied could have terminated pregnancies through legal abortion with-out parental consent, more than half chose to involve their mothers in the problem. Among whites, girls who planned to re-lease the baby for adoption were most likely to have a mother involved. Among blacks, it was those who planned to have an abortion. White girls who planned to keep their babies were more likely to turn to the baby's father for support than to their own mothers. Those girls who viewed themselves as com-petent tended to seek help less. Those who involved their moth-ers were more likely to experience conflict, but it is not clear whether this was cause or effect.

6 ◎◎◎◎◎◎◎◎◎◎◎◎◎◎◎

Substance Abuse

◎◎◎◎◎◎◎◎◎◎◎◎◎◎◎

Observers of social norms have acknowledged that, for many years, experimentation with tobacco and alcohol has been a part of many adolescents' development. The pattern of involvement with illicit drugs, however, is sharply different in our times today. Casual trial of soft (less severely addictive or harmful) drugs is so widespread that it is no longer a strong indicator of major pathology.

The number of persons, including teenagers, making serious and sustained use of drugs has required development of new treatment methods as a response to what has been called an epidemic of drug use in news reports. The implications to our society are frightening: In 1971, New York City statistics listed heroin as the major cause of death in males aged fifteen to

thirty-five. Other drugs may have serious and long lasting effects. Blunted or inappropriate emotionality, increased tendencies toward gratification of impulsive wishes, and temporary or sustained loss of some cognitive abilities are some of
these. Knowledge of potential effects of drug use clearly has
little deterrent value to the serious user.

Developments in treatment have not kept up with this
spreading problem. Hospitalization or outpatient dynamic
psychotherapy has not been notably successful. Modifications
in approach, some of which are described in this chapter, had to
be developed. Although we are a long way from being confident
of our chances of success with the individual addict, some progress has been made.

There are several possible reasons why teenagers try out
these substances and still other reasons why they continue their
use. Initial use may relate to peer relations. A youngster may
try a cigarette, a drink of beer or wine, or share a marihuana
joint in a group. Peer pressure, fear of exclusion, and the excitement of doing what many parents forbid all operate to support
experimentation. Another factor is parental usage. Adolescent
usage of alcohol and tobacco is greater in those youngsters
whose parents make regular use of these substances. This is also
true for teenagers who are significant users. Their parents often
have serious drug and alcohol problems. Parents who abuse substances and warn their children against usage are offering them a
convenient and effective way of expressing defiance. The teenager can show negativism by doing what is forbidden and express a reaction to a perceived parental "double standard." One
may speculate that, for these youngsters, serious substance
abuse may additionally represent imitation of parents, a behav-
ior-modeling process that seems to go on even during periods of
opposition and defiance. Perhaps some parents, sensing that
they are being imitated, express mixed feelings about this by an
inconsistent disciplinary response to their children's abuse.
Some parents accept abuse of alcohol or marihuana, thankful
the problem is not heroin. For these or other reasons, parents
manifest considerable difficulty in effectively disciplining their
substance-abusing children.

Following experimentation, other motivations that support continued use may emerge. These include short-lived escape from depression or anxious thoughts or situations. For some youngsters whose ego adjustment is shaky, use of chemicals can come to provide relief from the threat of breakdown. Alternately, the youngster may enjoy the experience of change to a mood more pleasant than the one he or she would have in facing reality. Having enjoyed this escape, repetition becomes easier. For others, use of a forbidden substance expresses anger and defiance of family or societal pressures.

A thorough assessment of the meaning of the abusing activity should be the starting point of treatment. Factors such as family dynamics and the youngster's age and social environment should be considered. Family factors in abuse include other members' use or abuse patterns and parental disciplinary skills. Absence of one parent is associated with greater risk of abuse, as well as other problems. The role of age results in different effects: A twelve-year-old's usage may begin largely as imitation; older teenagers' use carries more overtones of defiance. Reinforcers for drug use should be understood. Special attention is advised to the situations that drug use enables the youngster to avoid or escape.

Motivation to change abuse patterns is rare in serious users. They may complain instead of other problems in their life, but make an insufficient connection between these difficulties and the causal problem of drug dependence. Several writers, such as Bratter, argue that the first step is to increase motivation for change; however, this task is not easily accomplished. Hospitalization may be the next step for persistently unmotivated abusers.

For serious drug abusers, confrontative treatment communities such as Daytop, are alternatives to hospitalization if serious withdrawal is not a problem. The confrontative approach is part of most drug treatment strategies, such as Bratter's. A few writers suggest that individual treatment can be effective if certain guidelines are followed. A necessary first step is relationship formation. Werkman and Bratter (in his discussion of individual treatment) present approaches to this. The therapist should be in a position (even if idealized by the patient) to use his or her influence to press the issue of stopping drug use.

The articles in this chapter show a diversity of recent approaches to substance abuse problems in our time. Because the extent of this problem still far exceeds treatment efforts, development of better methods remains an urgent priority. It is hoped that critical examination of these interventions will stimulate exploration and improvements in treatment methods.

Treatment Recommendations Based on a Classification System

AUTHORS: S. Proskauer and R. S. Rolland

PRECIS: Three broad types of drug users and their treatment

INTRODUCTION: The authors feel that in today's society, drug use represents an adaptive defensive response, with drug reliance ranging from mild and transient interest to characterological dependence. This article presents several prescriptive options based on a psychodynamic assessment of the severity of usage as well as whether drug abuse should be considered the primary problem.

The three broad categories Proskauer and Rolland distinguish are experimental, depressive, and characterological drug users. For many adolescents, drug use, rarer in times past, is now a common, peer-accepted way of expressing oneself, showing defiance from parents and authorities. Experimental drug use of these teenagers is transient and benefits are short-lived. Peer pressures can get them to experiment, but not to use drugs steadily. Their social and emotional adaptation is generally good. It is best to avoid calling this type of youngster a drug abuser. It could overstate the role of drugs and provoke overly strong countermeasures by the adolescent. It can also raise excessive concern about the youngsters' self-concept.

A major preoccupation of depressive drug users is relief from negative feelings, such as depression and despair. Drugs, if easily available, may be employed as an easy escape. The depressive feature may be less visible and requires a careful assessment. Alienation from parents, few opportunities to acquire recognition based on present achievements, gender identity problems, and a deprived environment can be contributors to this picture.

Characterological drug users show problematic histories and major personality difficulties. Ego lacunae, needs for outside controls, and an urgent need to avoid distress are seen, together with psychological addiction. Rather than a release, drugs seem to fill in for their personal deficits. This severity is one way of distinguishing this group from the previous category.

TREATMENT METHOD: The experimental user's drug use is usually incorporated within a generally healthy period of experimentation, and treatment for drug use is not needed. A trusted adviser is often helpful.

It helps to educate depressive drug users about the escape function and neurotic self-defeating use of drugs on a specific-incident basis. It is hoped that they can still respond to suggestions and comments relating to their possible future. Peer supports through youth groups, skill and activity programs, as well as psychotherapy exploring depressive elements can be useful.

Insight therapy being unpromising, a mixture of assistance measures may help characterological drug users. The clinic therapist can support the patient's efforts to obtain help, especially at a self-help drug rehabilitation program. These DAYTOP type centers offer peer support and opportunities to obtain self-esteem by rebuilding one's life. However, living outside the supportive environment is viewed as threatening, and the supportive therapist should expect relapses.

COMMENTARY: This survey helps to remind us that although drug abuse is a diagnostic category, much more information is necessary to react appropriately to the adolescent's drug problem. Also prominent is the culturally modern view of drug experimentation as a comparatively minor episode for many teens, likely to be superseded by more socially positive activity.

SOURCE: Proskauer, S., and Rolland, R. S. "Youth Who Use Drugs: Psychodynamic Diagnosis and Treatment Planning." *Journal of the American Academy of Child Psychiatry*, 1973, *12*(1), 32-47.

Establishing the Therapeutic Alliance by Reducing Conflicts of Values

AUTHOR: S. Werkman

PRECIS: Strengthening the therapeutic alliance by approaching the adolescent through shared interests and values

INTRODUCTION: With the adolescent patient, the presenting problems frequently represent a direct assault on the values of the older generation, which are often those of the therapist as well. Drug use is one of the most difficult examples of these value conflicts. Differences in values between therapists and their adolescent patients can interfere with the therapeutic process. Issues about which there are differences include the significance of education, work, and achievement; sexual morality; and materialistic philosophy. An additional problem is that many adolescents reject the notion of solving problems through therapy because it involves accepting the passive role of patient. They prefer to seek their own solutions actively through sensitivity groups, informal rap sessions, and drug experimentation. The problems that propel adolescents into treatment are often "now" problems for which they want an immediate solution. The therapist can be hard put to compete with the immediate solutions available through drug use.

CASE HISTORY: The patient was an eighteen-year-old boy with a history of drug abuse who had recently made a suicide attempt. His father, at whose request he had come to therapy, was a successful businessman. The boy presented with long hair and a beard, wearing dirty, tattered clothing. He was initially hostile and defensive, but after some banter about a book which he was carrying, he was willing to discuss the suicide attempt. Discussion of his musical interests was used as a bridge to discussing attitudes toward his family. He subsequently expressed a fear that the therapist would attempt to impose his values on him and that his acceptance of those values would lead to a boring and meaningless life, like that of his father. He became more involved in therapy when the therapist was able to feed his interest in transcendental meditation by putting him into a light hypnotic trance. As therapy progressed, it became clear that major problems to be overcome included lack of trust and fears concerning close personal relationships and severe inhibition of aggression and competitiveness.

COMMENTARY: The author points out that therapists need to carefully examine their values in relation to those of the youths with whom they work and to consider whether there is sufficient overlap to support a therapeutic relationship. He suggests that one way to reach patients like the one described is through their interest in nonrational experience and that techniques that involve altered states of consciousness can be an effective means of capturing their attention for therapeutic work. He does not describe the actual course of therapy, but his orientation is clearly psychoanalytic. An alternative, behavioral approach like systematic desensitization, described elsewhere in this book, might provide the immediate success experiences necessary to sustaining the treatment relationship. This approach has the advantage that the adolescent can actively use it to solve other problems as they occur. Family interviews could have been used to clarify parental values, perhaps bringing to light ambiguities and highlighting parental behaviors reinforcing immaturity.

SOURCE: Werkman, S. "Value Confrontations Between Therapists and Their Adolescent Patients." *American Journal of Orthopsychiatry*, 1974, *44*, 337-344.

Individual Treatment for
Unmotivated Abusers

AUTHOR: T. E. Bratter

PRECIS: A four-stage program to assist recovery of effective
functioning in the alienated user

INTRODUCTION: Bratter's criteria for drug abuse are when
drug use clearly occupies much of an adolescent's thinking or
when it replaces social or intellectual functioning. The steps
outlined here derive from work with the children of affluent
suburban families. Typical findings are fathers overinvolved in
work or outside activities and uninvolved in home life, where
the mother is overly controlling, either by threat or by entice-
ment. Generally, parents are exceedingly permissive. Bratter rejects traditional psychotherapeutic as well as nondirective procedures because they are not appropriate to deal with the
self-destructive aspects of this pattern.

TREATMENT METHOD: Bratter describes four stages of treatment. The first is *establishing a therapeutic alliance.* The therapist describes and explains obstacles to involvement in treatment. Suspicion, for example, is the adolescent's habit, and no
wonder, considering some of the illegal activities often accompanying drug use. Thus a therapist shows an understanding of
the patient's world. The therapist also assumes parent-surrogate
functions, including opposition to drugs. One's opposition to
the self-destructive aspect of drugs should be clear. Adolescents
are often testing at this point. Bratter is one of many who treat
testing as expressing a genuine need to know where limits and
boundaries are. Adolescents come to feel secure by learning the
strength of the therapist's responses. Another relationship-building step is to encourage phone calls any time there is a serious
chance of acting out. For the patient, this is a first step toward
anticipating problems.

The second stage is *forced behavioral change.* This is done
to reach a lower, less debilitating level of drug use. The thera-

pist's limit setting is atypically active, with arguing, even demanding that drug use be reduced. If this is not carried out, the patient has shown no rational self-interest and further steps are taken, including calling in parents to discuss whether the abuser can be treated at home. Bratter's experience is that calling in parents is beneficial when indicated.

Third is *reorientation and reconstruction of behavior.* Through pointing out the existence of freedom of choice and self-control options, the therapist displays the patient's full responsibility for his or her behavior. The patient is challenged to try to exercise control over negative responses, such as drug use. Clarification of one's own goals is a target, along with how future goals conflict with past activities. Whether there is genuine desire to change is discussed. The therapist's objective is to foster the sense that present solutions are inadequate and only continuous self-searching can lead to new choices.

The fourth stage is *growth and development.* As self-inquiry is accepted as valuable, the therapist helps strengthen this process by assigning tasks, such as writing goals and contracting to reach them. The therapist can begin to act more like a consultant/adviser at this stage, helping the patient to think about planning. The therapist is not deterred from a positive, realistic opinion about the adolescent's potential to achieve. If there is success, limited praise should be accompanied by the clear understanding that this is not a resting point. If goals are not reached, however, the standards can still be praised while lack of effort is actively deplored.

Bratter has sometimes actively intervened in the patient's outside situation to secure a potential benefit. He has argued together with the patient at schools and courts, strengthening his alliance with the patient's positive strivings. In doing so, he also models assertive responses to local institutions, another skill commonly lacking in his patients.

COMMENTARY: This article is a thoughtful review of several treatment issues in cases of minimally responsive patients. He recognizes the need for much energy and time and rapid response to adolescent crises. His is a reasoned response to the problems of limit setting in drug abuse. In setting demands for reduction of use, he avoids unrealistic demands for abstinence and hopefully contributes to internal conflict in the patient. Bratter's follow-up data indicate that he has helped this high-risk population. Of sixty-four patients followed up, forty-five were working or in school and thirty-five were completely drug free.

SOURCE: Bratter, T. E. "Treating Alienated, Unmotivated Drug-Abusing Adolescents." *American Journal of Psychotherapy*, 1973, 27(4), 585-598.

An Open Group Confrontation Approach with Affluent Users

AUTHOR: T. E. Bratter

PRECIS: Use of therapist and peer feedback to reverse abandonment of personal responsibility

INTRODUCTION: This approach has developed out of a wealthy community's concern with youngsters' drug use. The use of drugs is conceptualized here as acting out of anger at a breakdown in the parental relationship. The program features easy entry into the group, a flexible format and time schedule, and therapist and peer focus on an individual in the "hot seat."

CASE HISTORY: Craig was one of three sons of a hardworking distant father and a mother who was mainly self-preoccupied. The mother was given to self-critical remarks and punitiveness when the boy failed to live up to her expectations. Craig seemed to be her favorite. Eight years of school problems began in the fourth grade, with eventual expulsion following Craig's refusal to accept an imposed suspension for suspected drug dealing. He had begun using his mother's various diet and sleeping pills, later progressing to hallucinogens. His parents showed considerable marital difficulties. Entering analysis at his parents' insistence, he increased abuse, leading to a recommendation of hospitalization.

He attended the group with friends one night, and treated the leader with anger and rudeness. He seemed to be displacing feelings about his father and expected peer support for this anti-authoritarian stance. The therapist, followed by the group, rejected his explanation that his excess drug abuse and antisocial behavior were due to mental illness. They attributed it to stupidity and the wish to provoke.

In the next session, when he finally agreed with this, he spoke of peoples' convictions that nothing good could any longer be expected of him. He seemed to want another chance in school, but no support by parents or local authorities was likely. The therapist, who also taught a university graduate psychology course, got the school to agree to grant credit should he pass. A no-drug contract requiring good attendance and performance was drawn up. When he smoked pot near the end, he had to negotiate with the school for a revised, *more* stringent contract, without any assistance by the therapist this time. He passed the course and returned to high school. He maintained an improved level of performance, interspersed with several serious episodes of self-defeating behavior. On the whole, however, the antisocial behavior was greatly reduced. He completed high school, moved to his own apartment, and was accepted at a good college.

TREATMENT METHOD: Open group therapy sessions dealing with drug problems are widely advertised. Attendance is entirely open to all. When adults attend, it seems to stimulate adolescents' activity; they use the meeting as a communication channel. Discussion in the meeting focuses on peoples' perception of reasons for drug abuse. The aim is to urge reduced usage, although no enforcement is attempted.

Confrontation is vigorous about the self-defeating aspects of drug use. There is discussion of peoples' inability to accept external standards; feelings of being labeled, rejected, and un-loved; and being seen as failures. One member tends to emerge as the focus of each meeting, receiving feedback from peers and therapists. The group presses for the abuser to accept sole re-sponsibility for the abuse and to make a commitment to change. Other group members are not permitted to act as advocates for the user. They may later act as assistants, monitoring or advising the user on his or her attempts to stop.

The therapist demonstrates concern by a high level of par-ticipation in the group. He states his commitment to drug-free living, his belief in the possibility of the users' self-rehabilita-tion, and his expectations of more progress than the adolescent wishes to promise. Especially noteworthy is the therapist's will-ingness, once he is convinced of motivation to change, to nego-tiate with schools and courts to obtain new chances for the im-proving youngster.

COMMENTARY: Bratter clearly describes a therapist-directed program that successfully engages unmotivated adolescents to examine their drug use. Both drug rehabilitation and psycho-therapeutic methods are used. The easy admission and accessi-bility of the group (four times weekly in different places in the town) enhance the program's appeal. The program leader should be familiar with group dynamics and encounter techniques, fan-tasy methods, and behavior contracting and be ready to re-spond to testing and backsliding.

SOURCE: Bratter, T. E. "Group Therapy with Affluent, Ali-enated, Adolescent Drug Users: A Reality Therapy and Con-frontation Approach." *Psychotherapy: Theory, Research and Practice,* 1972, *9*(4), 308-313.

Family Contracting

AUTHORS: L. W. Frederiksen, J. O. Jenkins, and C. R. Carr

PRECIS: Decreased drug abuse by contracted change of non-drug-related behavior

INTRODUCTION: Contingency contracting has been successful in treatment of many behaviors, including drug abuse. The client and the family agree on which rewards will follow certain specific behaviors. The therapist usually acts to assist all parties in maintaining and improving their adherence to the contractual agreement. A problem with directly treating drug abuse is the difficulty of checking whether change has actually occurred. Other undesirable behaviors could be primary change targets, according to the authors. These might be more reliably, easily, and inexpensively monitored. Also, decreased drug use may be of limited duration in an adolescent with continued social or family problems. In this study, the major focus was on deteriorated family communication.

CASE HISTORY: A seventeen-year-old male had been arrested for drug possession twice within a brief period of time. He admitted to three years' daily use of many drugs, orally and by injection. He had completed high school and was unemployed. He was in a nonvoluntary drug treatment program. He was living with his parents, who came for interviews with him. During the first interview it became clear that drug use started when the family relationship declined. He maintained usage because it avoided family problems, he got peer reinforcement, and it felt good.

TREATMENT METHOD: The family agreed to three treatment goals: improved relationships, the son's lessened drug use, and his need for career-oriented activity. The treatment program did not, however, address drug use. Instead, a contingency contract was constructed and implemented to cover the following tasks: activities to help him get ready for vocational school; using and taking care of the family car; allowance; and curfew.

Family members prepared the contract in four sessions. All were urged to raise problems, express their view of desired behaviors, and clarify what the reinforcers were to be. (Although the contract is not detailed in the article, the task list gives clues to problem areas, privileges, and required behaviors.) Next, the sessions focused primarily on how well members were carrying out the agreement. Confusions or poorly negotiated parts of the contract could be changed. Family members were made aware they might be called at any time to find out how the contract was going.

TREATMENT RESULTS: The contract was carried out successfully. Parents' self-ratings on a parent-child happiness scale, markedly low at the outset, improved as soon as the contract was in force. Interestingly, the son's happiness self-ratings improved even more quickly, while the contract was being negotiated. Drug use, checked by random lab screening and family report, was described as markedly reduced. It remained at that level at one-year follow-up.

COMMENTARY: This program applies the well-tested principle of strengthening desirable behaviors that are incompatible with negative ones, such as drug use. Work toward the agreed-upon goals (car care, school-related activities, family negotiation, and attention to curfew) were significantly opposite to heavy use of drugs. The son was apparently motivated to change but needed a structured intervention and support, which this program provided. The son perceived negotiation training of all parties as beneficial, as may be inferred from his self-ratings. This approach is worth considering when the abuser shows some motivation and the family is willing to help.

SOURCE: Frederiksen, L. W., Jenkins, J. O., and Carr, C. R. "Indirect Modification of Adolescent Drug Abuse Using Contingency Contracting." *Journal of Behavior Therapy and Experimental Psychiatry*, 1976, *7*, 377-378.

Crisis-Oriented Psychotherapy

AUTHOR: R. A. Geist

PRECIS: Providing a therapeutic dependence in initial stages of treatment as an alternative to drug dependence

INTRODUCTION: When a teenager is in an aggravated situation, such as a personal crisis, one has the chance to see behaviors and feelings that might take years to emerge within a therapeutic relationship. The author developed a crisis center, to which youngsters come voluntarily, in a high school. They show a pattern of exaggeration of some common adolescent problems, including severe depressive, even nihilistic moods, sexual acting out, usually within a minimal emotional relationship, a passive response to the normal home and school situations, and behavioral and drug-induced activity reactive to a sense of time passing. They also show a need to excessively trust and feel cared for by peers (while denying evidence of rejection by them).

Philosophically and in behavior, there is a search for antidotes or responses to reality pressures. This may stem from two early sources—feeling unprotected from familial aggressive or sexual pressures and feeling lack of familial nurture. Geist feels that many adolescents take drugs largely in response to persistent feelings of defenselessness and vulnerability. These feelings make acceptance of oneself as separate even more difficult.

TREATMENT METHOD: The treatment relationship should be viewed as a "transitional object," helping the drug abuser to achieve a separation from drug dependence. This is a first goal, and to support it the therapist is available for extra appointments at critical, needy periods. Missed appointments are less challenged at first, in the interest of maximizing positive contact.

Strong pressures by the therapist to cease drug use may not be advisable. When the relationship with the therapist is more secure, this effort may begin. The patient's capability of handling problems in better ways can be explored. Similarly, within a stronger relationship the issue of missed appointments or lateness can be raised.

Better results may be achieved by responding to the person's active strategies rather than by exploring passive defenses. For example, the "automatic opposite" (counterdependent) pattern of one youngster's behavior was examined. The suggestion that this was just as dependent a reaction was picked up quickly.

A crisis of choice (drugs versus relationships, especially with the therapist) can be expected. This signals the adolescent's increasing sense of lacks in his life. Vulnerability, leading to a "need" to depend on others or on drugs, becomes an issue. A therapist may find that a concept of separateness with less dependence is still difficult to tolerate.

Issues of dependency may manifest themselves in sexual relationships. These should be explored to understand if they represent acting out related to treatment or additional "transitional" relationships helping to achieve separation. The dependency, intimacy, and needs aspects of such relationships may be mentioned. This is to assist the youngster in understanding the place and limitations of such events in meeting his or her felt needs. With more realistic expectations, perhaps future attachments may be more stable.

COMMENTARY: Two common problems in treating drug abusers are low motivation and poor relating. In a crisis model, the therapist intervenes when motivation is temporarily high so that some beginnings can perhaps be made. Allowing exaggerated dependence may help a sustained effort to be maintained. Assisting legitimate independence strivings may happen late in treatment. The author does not devote much space to any problems of reducing dependence upon the therapist.

An additional complicating factor is the difficulty in tolerating the passage of time. The author reminds us that patients (and some drug treatment philosophies) treat personality change as easier than most personality theorists view it. The slowness of change must be accepted by the therapist so that the difficulties in maturing can be revealed to the patient.

SOURCE: Geist, R. A. "Some Observations on Adolescent Drug Use: Therapeutic Implications." *Journal of the American Academy of Child Psychiatry*, 1974, *13*, 54-71.

Paradoxical Intervention in an Atypical Abuser

AUTHOR: G. Morelli

PRECIS: Reduction of drug and alcohol consumption in an overconsuming female

INTRODUCTION: Paradoxical intention is a specific technique used with a variety of problem behaviors. Developed by Viktor Frankl, it is often used with complaints of behaviors that evoke strong fears. This case applies the procedure to a different maladaptive behavior, substance abuse, not evoking such feelings. The patient is verbally encouraged to do what he or she claims to be trying to avoid—to fail the test, to get very tense or hysterically upset, and so forth. This is directed at the anticipatory anxiety. Frequently when patients attempt to respond, they find themselves having difficulty in doing the feared disastrous act and anxiety quickly lessens.

CASE HISTORY: Although this eighteen-year-old female originally was referred for obesity, a major drug and alcohol abuse problem was soon singled out for treatment. She reported a two-year history of use of amphetamines, hallucinogenics, stimulants, depressants, and moderate to excessive alcohol use. She had a good academic record from high school and was initially seen in her last semester there. Initial treatment centered on weight loss, and in fact she lost 14 pounds from her original 169 (she was five foot one). Over the summer, using drugs and alcohol as well, she gained it back and more. By midterm in her first college semester, her grade average was D.

At that point the therapist focused on substance abuse, using paradoxical intention. When she described her extent of use, the response was surprise that so little had been used. The therapist suggested that she take much more, naming specific types and amounts of drugs. When she replied that to do this would lead to lateness, missed assignments, and failure, he answered that he expected nothing to be handed in, that she could miss all classes and leave school. He urged her to consume drugs, despite her surprise at this. Whenever she mentioned substance abuse, he reminded her she could do more. He did, however, express positive responses to her reports of being increasingly on time and doing work. Results began practically at once, with reduced use of drugs and alcohol. Occasional marihuana use and one or two weekend beers became her new pattern. She moved away from her dorm to avoid the life-style there, which she felt to be not serious enough. Follow-up at midterm and end of term in her second semester showed no increase in drug use. Her second semester average was B+.

COMMENTARY:The author suggests that the common response to an adolescent's drug use—it is bad, against the law, and such—avoids the fact of direct consequence of the abuse. The patient may prefer to focus on the defiance and rule-breaking aspects, showing opposition to parental or societal norms. Morelli shifts the issue to whether drug use helps to reach the patient's own goals. This patient showed several characteristics that led to paradoxical intention as a treatment of choice. She was motivated, having been in therapy for several months, and had a good prior academic record. She was not described as being heavily identified with the drug culture. This technique may not apply to the unmotivated abuser, but it is worth considering when the patient has strongly felt goals.

SOURCE: Morelli, G. "Paradoxical Intention: A Case Study of an Effective Method of Treating Alcoholism and Drug Abuse." *Psychology*, 1978, *15*, 57-59.

Using Paraprofessionals with Hard-to-Reach Families of Abusers

AUTHORS: J. D. Teicher, R. D. Sinay, and J. S. Stumphauzer

PRECIS: Employing paraprofessionals in applications of learning theory to family treatment of teenage drinking

INTRODUCTION: Two major innovations are reported here. First, there is the use of a family behavior therapy model with teenage drinkers. This work is based on Stumphauzer's earlier research, showing that alcohol abuse tends to be very strongly modeled and reinforced. Rarely is punishment or effort to limit its use observed. Second, the use of paraprofessionals is described. This was in response to the fact that after discharge from a crisis treatment program, teenagers were not coming for the aftercare phase. Experienced minority group community workers were selected to learn how to conduct a behavioral program in the home.

TREATMENT METHOD: The community workers received weekly training sessions for six months, beginning with learning theory and family contracting. Two manuals, one on parenting and one by Stumphauzer on behavior therapy principles, were among the teaching materials. Behavior therapy sessions were also observed and reviewed. The training phase included treatment of three families.

Families were seen with the following format, which varied for each family in the number of sessions required for each stage: (1) *Initial approach,* in which the paraprofessional met with the parent or teenager. The goal was information gathering and a mutual decision to work together; (2) *Assessment,* in which problems, possible reinforcers, and ways of measuring behavior (such as behavior cards to record activities) were considered; (3) *First contract,* which was worked out among the adolescent, parents, and paraprofessional. To increase the chances of rapid initial reinforcement and success, a simple example was selected; (4) *Revision and expansion of the contract,* in which more complex bargains in areas of substance abuse, school, and family problems were explored with contracts. The goal in family sessions was improved interactions and a shift from punishment to praise and reward where appropriate; (5) *Separation from treatment,* which was accomplished as contracts were made on the outside with less help.

CASE HISTORY: Twelve-year old Chavo's major problems were drinking and missing school. The first contract, for four weeks, called for him to attend school while sober. Each successful day, he received time with the paraprofessional and fifty cents to spend. By the fourth week, he was collecting every day. The second contract then focused on his gang activity and called for reinforced activity incompatible with gang behavior. For example, he had to regularly call home when out, spend more time at home, and, of course, go to school. He was allowed to earn Fridays out until midnight. By the fourth week, Chavo was able to fulfill all conditions.

COMMENTARY: The success of this program is emphasized by the fact that the parents and teachers who cooperated began to apply the contracting techniques with other children. Selection and training of the paraprofessionals is a critical element for the success of such a program. Not all potential workers will complete training successfully. This pilot project illustrates the importance and the difficulty of recruiting community workers who are sensitive to differing cultural values and to the resistance to admission of problems shown by minority group families.

SOURCE: Teicher, J. D., Sinay, R. D., and Stumphauzer, J. S. "Training Community-Based Paraprofessionals as Behavior Therapists with Families of Alcohol-Abusing Adolescents." *American Journal of Psychiatry,* 1976, *133*(7), 847-850.

A Group Consultation Procedure to
Change Attitudes Toward Drugs

AUTHORS: L. D. Tashjian and L. H. Crabtree, Jr.

PRECIS: An educative, large group process model to foster dialogue

INTRODUCTION: The authors, members of a drug consultation group, acknowledge several problems hindering the effectiveness of various drug counseling programs for teenagers. For example, feeling scolded or lectured, teenagers invoke a habit of "tuning out." Media material, often quite graphic, can be titillating and enhance the likelihood of experimentation. Ex-addicts' presentations are also frequently used. However, teenagers may adapt a denial pose—"I couldn't be that dumb," "I can stop any time I want to," and so forth. The authors believe that several other problems hinder awareness of the problem associated with drug abuse. The news of serious physical or psychological effects seem unimpressive to this audience, who may have heard reports of scientific ambivalence or friends' accounts of wonderful trips. Further, drug use is often a key to joining the group, doing something forbidden, separating from the adult environment. These assumptions, plus one other, underlie the procedures used by this group. The additional assumption is that suspicion, splitting, and hostility are as prominent between adolescent subgroupings as they are between teens and adults.

TREATMENT METHOD: The goals of the consultation are (1) offering nondrug alternatives to users and increasing likelihood of continued abstinence in nonusers; (2) increasing positive feelings about oneself in the world by decreasing subgroup and teen-adult polarizations, to decrease the alienating factors in the agency where the intervention is taking place; and (3) to set a tone in the visited facility that fosters more dialogue and sharing of experiences.

At a meeting of fifty to one hundred students, no school personnel are present and confidentiality is explained. The "staff" number about a dozen. Some of the staff are currently patients in an adolescent treatment center. After a brief opening, questions are invited. At this time, inquiries may be trivial or provocative, but all are written on the blackboard. While most of the staff goes to sit or mingle with the audience, the questioners are invited on stage. Some challenging emerges, which is not responded to, deliberately raising tension and hostility. The usual result is a strong attack, representing a polarized, entrenched position on drugs. This is followed by the emergence of subgroups clearly committed to opposite positions. Shouting and arguing, but not listening, are frequent. At this point the first intervention, to develop listening, is made. People are told to speak only in the first person, making personal assertions. Alternately, the group process is confronted, with prejudice, isolation, hostility, and the use of poses to cover fear of presenting one's true nature revealed as the major themes. The goal of this step is reduction of splitting and animosity by developing active participation in the discussion. After this step is reached, sixty to ninety minutes into the presentation, there is a division into three small groups, moderated by staff. Personal concerns such as belonging, obstacles to being genuine, dealing with inner contradictions, estrangement, and alienation are discussed far more than drugs. Pro- and antidrug students are thus sharing common perspectives and feelings. In a warmer, more responsive atmosphere, this active investment enhances the notion that one has something worth sharing.

TREATMENT RESULTS: Summary and conclusions from a dozen consultations are that the program has been well received, with no consequent problems or negative reactions. All places have issued return invitations. No evaluation of subsequent drug use was done, and the general attitude toward marihuana is apparently unaltered. However, peer attitudes against harder drugs is more pronounced, and nonusers and minimal users are more confidently able to refrain. Moreover, increased dialogue and cooperation have been commonly observed, with some groups being spontaneously set up to continue an issue raised at the consultation.

COMMENTARY: A noteworthy feature of this approach is the preference for shifting away from the drug-informative intervention to the issues of relatedness and more personal concerns common to all. The presence as staff of adolescents in treatment, who can be part of a common voice with the staff but also join with the concerns of their fellow teens, is no doubt quite stimulating. We include this article because of its use of group dynamics in attacking this specific problem of drug use. This procedure may be helpful in similar agency situations where a group is sharply divided on another issue, apparently without hope of getting together. The sequence described here—developing polarity and anxiety, exploring defensive distancing, and finally discovering common issues—may be worth consideration.

If this program could be carried further, two steps might be taken. The first would be evaluation of any change in drug use or major incidents in the facility. A second step might be to help the facility lend some institutional supports to student-led activities stemming from these consultations. One such example is a drug emergency group started by students at one school.

SOURCE: Tashjian, L. D., and Crabtree, L. H., Jr. "A Group Method of Altering Adolescent Attitudes Toward Drug Use." *Psychotherapy: Theory, Research and Practice,* 1972, *9,* 314-316.

Additional Readings

Caroff, P., Lieberman, F., and Gottesfeld, M. "The Drug Problem: Treating Preaddictive Adolescents." *Social Casework,* 1970, *51,* 527-532.

The authors' work was with youngsters referred for school problems but who were found to have significant drug involvement. Their parents' lack of clear prohibition meant that the support for their attempts to control their behavior was lacking.

From the point of referral, the parents were advised that this represented a crisis situation. The parents often felt sympathy with their children's protest issues and counterculture investment. They were told that effective, good parenting required prohibition of illegal use of substances. Their commitment to this was required for participation. Parents received much support for this effort. Emergency contact by telephone was available. The therapist's conviction of the worth of the no-drug stance was essential. Talk about drugs was not allowed after the initial phase of entry into treatment. The retelling of drug experiences was observed to reinforce drug use.

Griffin, J. B., Jr. "Some Psychodynamic Considerations in the Treatment of Drug Abuse in Early Adolescence." *Journal of the American Academy of Child Psychiatry,* 1981, *20,* 159-166.

Drug abuse among early adolescents was sharply curtailed by a plan developed by concerned parents. The plan featured an effective approach to the youngsters based on sound understanding of their psychodynamic and subcultural issues. Although drug use was fun, aided escape from problems, and got peer support, in the author's view it produced alienation, not age-appropriate separation, and pseudomaturation, not independent growth. Parents formed a group to discuss the problem, which helped reduce their guilt and anger. Parents learned that drugs could weaken ego control of emerging adolescent impulses. Action guidelines were developed. Parents informed the children of their stand against all drug use. They offered supervised social alternative activities, rather than focus on their anger and punitive urges. Some of this anger was channeled into political action, resulting in the closing of several head shops. Guidelines at home were more strictly enforced. The younger adolescents' angry reactions to this were short-lived, and most later expressed appreciation for being made to stop. Acceptance of this was easier when they saw parents' greater anger toward local drug suppliers.

Huberty, C., and Huberty, D. J. "Treating the Parents of Adolescent Drug Abusers." *Contemporary Drug Problems,* 1976 (Winter), 573–592.

This program does not deal directly with adolescents, but with their parents, whose marriage is often too strained to allow their drug-abusing child to return. Parents require some "selfish time" to restore their relationship before they can offer real help to their child. The Hubertys use three approaches: information on chemical dependency and the family problems it typically causes; exploration of family roles and values that make up the family constellation; and confrontation. The couple's denial of the extent of the problem is common. Other times they may be split on how to respond. Both may be ambivalent, with one common result being that the partners take extreme opposing views that they cannot reconcile. Parents are taught and urged to work together to set and enforce limits. Support is provided for the efforts they make, their attempts to deal with current challenges, and their efforts to rebuild communications through exercises.

Kolvin, I. " 'Aversive Imagery' Treatment in Adolescents." *Behavior Research and Therapy*, 1967, *5*, 245-248.

A nonphysical aversive procedure was used with a fifteen-year-old male with a seven-year history of gasoline sniffing. This was his principal recreation. He had passed out from sniffing, reporting hallucinations. In residential treatment for the educationally handicapped, he was a husky, pleasant boy. A list of most disliked experiences was obtained. He learned to relax and visualize pleasant images of sniffing. When observably involved, the noxious images were verbally presented, disrupting the pleasure. Sessions of two to four trials were held five days a week. A total of twenty sessions was held. He reported discomfort early on and soon stated he had lost the urge to use gasoline. Follow-up at thirteen months showed no relapse. In this article, Kolvin describes the application of this same approach to a fourteen-year-old fetishist.

Lamontagne, Y., Beausejour, R., Annable, L., and Tetreault, L. "Alpha and EMG Feedback Training in the Prevention of Drug Abuse." *Canadian Psychiatric Association Journal*, 1977, *22*, 301-310.

In a controlled experiment, college students had twelve

thirty-minute training sessions under different conditions. The students who received EMG training who were considered moderate users of drugs (six to thirteen times monthly) lowered their drug use and maintained this at one- and three-month follow-up. Heavy users showed a nonsignificant trend to reduced use. Results for the alpha-wave training group were not as positive. No change of usage was observed for alcohol or cigarette use. EMG is suggested as a drug preventive procedure. We think this could be incorporated into a wide variety of programs and should appeal to adolescents.

Stumphauzer, J. "Learning to Drink: Adolescents and Alcohol." *Addictive Behaviors*, 1980, *5*, 277-283.

The author clarifies the learning and reinforcement elements in teenage drinking and points out implications for treatment. This data was collected on psychiatrically hospitalized adolescents. Presence of friends who were drinking was the most important antecedent factor. There was little regard for the potential harmful effects or the illegality of the drinking. Reinforcing consequences included rapid change of feeling peer approval and, surprisingly, parental approval. Sometimes parents expressed the reaction that drinking was preferable to drug use. Recall of how much they drank or how drunk they were was also pleasurable. Behavioral therapy of alcohol abuse is based on analysis and treatment of each of these antecedent, consumption-inducing variables. Reports of this approach are chiefly with adults. Work on modification for adolescent drinkers is needed.

Stybel, L. J. "Psychotherapeutic Options in the Treatment of Child and Adolescent Hydrocarbon Inhalers." *American Journal of Psychotherapy*, 1977, *31*, 525-532.

Hydrocarbon inhaling is still found among adolescents, though its popularity may have waned somewhat. Stybel distinguishes three classes of severity of abuse, with treatment options for each. His findings suggest that 75 percent are *social* sniffers, who see this as a group activity. Identifying with a new group or discovering alternate pleasurable activities usually stops the sniffing. Fifteen percent of users are *moderate* sniffers (about four to nineteen times per month). Their use could become greater; so intervention is necessary. Group therapy, parent training, and change of behavior consequences for sniffing have been reported to be effective. *Chronic* users, about 10 percent of the group, are older and signs of significant deterioration are present. They may present like simple schizophrenics, and hospitalization may be necessary. Case examples are provided.

7

Suicidal Behavior

Adolescent suicide is a major public health problem. Suicide is one of the leading causes of death in the adolescent years; and taking into account the likelihood that many suicides are disguised as accidents, it could even be the number one cause. If one considers that the ratio of attempted suicides to completed suicides may be as high as a hundred to one (I. B. Weiner, "Psychopathology in Adolescence," in J. Adelson, Ed., *Handbook of Adolescent Psychology*, New York: Wiley, 1980), the problem assumes even greater proportions.

Although many adolescent suicides appear to be impulsive acts in response to trivial problems, there are generally chronic predisposing factors (L. Wright, A. B. Schafer, and G. Solomons, *Encyclopedia of Pediatric Psychology*, Baltimore: Univer-

351

sity Park Press, 1979). Those who make suicide attempts often come from families in which there is parental indifference or even an active wish to be rid of the child. Parents may be highly demanding and unrealistic in their expectations. There is frequently a history of significant loss, particularly loss of a parent; and depression is a likely concomitant of suicidal behavior. The suicide attempter often has failed to establish or maintain significant peer relationships outside the home. For the young person already in such a precarious position, the developmental tasks of adolescence may prove overwhelming, and stresses like chronic illness, school failure, or additional loss through death or separation may lead to intolerable feelings of anxiety and depression.

Early detection of suicide potential is an important aspect of prevention. This requires a knowledge of predisposing factors and precipitating causes as well as an openness to subtle communication of thought and feeling. Physicians, teachers, guidance counselors, and others who work with young people may recognize the potential for suicide in a youth who is not otherwise involved with mental health services. With supportive consultation, they can make appropriate referrals. The alert therapist may also see suicide potential in patients who have come to him or her with other presenting problems. Pfeffer (see Additional Readings) has gone so far as to recommend that every child evaluated psychiatrically should be assessed for early warning signs of suicide.

The adolescent who attempts suicide is often making a last attempt to get help with what seems to him or her to be an intolerable problem (I. B. Weiner, "Psychopathology in Adolescence," in J. Adelson (Ed.), *Handbook of Adolescent Psychology,* New York: Wiley, 1980). Usually they have been struggling for some time with concerns they cannot resolve. The way in which their cry for help is responded to will influence the likelihood of future attempts.

A suicide attempt represents an immediate crisis that requires an appropriate therapeutic response. The seriousness of the attempt and the degree of continued risk must be assessed; precipitating stresses must be determined and alleviated where possible; and a period of protective hospitalization may be necessary so that information can be gathered and family and community supports can be mobilized.

Long-term treatment is usually indicated for the more chronic difficulties that predispose a particular youth to suicidal behavior. Family pathology such as lack of parental involvement and poor communication along with individual symptoms like depression, low self-esteem, and poor impulse control all require attention. Skills deficits resulting in academic failure or social isolation are important targets, and manifestations of serious psychopathology must also be treated. A significant problem is the patient's overwhelming sense of isolation and aloneness. The therapeutic relationship offers some relief, but treatment planning should also be directed toward mobilizing other significant interpersonal relationships as bulwarks against such feelings.

The therapist who works with suicidal adolescents must be capable of both firmness and flexibility, especially if treatment is carried out on an outpatient basis (J. A. Motto, "Treatment and Management of Suicidal Adolescents," *Psychiatric Opinion,* 1975, *12,* 14-20). Needs for emotional support or help in resolving a crisis may not coincide with scheduled appointments. The client is likely to be demanding, manipulative, and difficult to engage in a relationship. The therapist must at times set firm limits on behavior (see Bratter in Additional Readings) and must also be flexible in accommodating to needs that cannot wait until the next appointment. The strong emotions aroused may lead to a desire on the part of the therapist for quick solutions, but as Hochberg (see Additional Readings) points out, therapy is a process of growth and development, and it rarely follows the therapist's timetable.

The articles presented in this chapter address both prevention and treatment of adolescent suicide. Most stress the need for a combination of approaches. Individual psychotherapy is clearly important in both prevention and treatment, but because of the importance of family dynamics in the predisposition to suicide, family therapy is frequently recommended as part of a comprehensive intervention plan. Behavioral techniques also play an important part in decreasing both suicidal ideation and behavior.

A Telephone Hotline for
Suicide Prevention

AUTHOR: H. C. Faigel

PRECIS: Presents causes, early warning signs, and an approach to prevention for adolescent suicide

INTRODUCTION: The true incidence of suicide among adolescents is not known, but experts agree that it has been increasing for a number of years. To prevent adolescent suicide, it is necessary to understand its causes, be familiar with early warning signs, and have a well-developed strategy for engaging those at risk in psychological treatment.

CAUSES OF ADOLESCENT SUICIDE: Faigel lists a number of salient causes of adolescent suicide. Depression resulting from personal loss through death or divorce of parents is a common problem in the at-risk group. The younger the child was at the time of loss, the greater the probable impact. Disturbed family relationships, ambivalence of the parents toward the child, economic distress, illness, and overly strict discipline are also common in the histories of suicide attempters.

PREDICTING SUICIDE ATTEMPTS: Common dangers signals that have been found useful in assessing the degree of risk include the following:

1. History of a previous attempt
2. Accident proneness
3. Recent death in the family
4. Recent disruption of the family
5. Repressed anger
6. Poor self-image
7. Anxieties about sexuality
8. Depression

PREVENTION: The prevention program described involves the

use of a telephone hotline in a large western city. The phone number was well publicized and phone coverage was available twenty-four hours a day, seven days a week. Therapists answering the phones were responsible for providing psychological first aid, assessing the suicide risk, and formulating a tentative treatment plan. Program effects are not detailed, but during a one-year period, there were sixteen hundred calls at night or on the weekend. Eighty-five of these were young people between the ages of eleven and twenty.

COMMENTARY: Faigel describes causes and early warning signs of adolescent suicide and suggests a telephone hotline as one way of making services accessible to the at-risk group. The average number of people served on any given evening by this hotline was about four or five. No data are presented on the dimensions of the at-risk group; so it is not possible to evaluate the extent to which the hotline succeeded in reaching them. It might be that an effective prevention program requires more than one way of gaining access to services. Whatever the method for establishing contact, however, it is also necessary to have clearly spelled out in advance the procedures for implementing follow-up treatment. Particularly important is the need for agreements with hospitals and other institutions providing emergency services to give such cases priority treatment.

SOURCE: Faigel, H. C. "Suicide Among Young Persons: A Review of Its Incidence and Causes, and Methods for Its Prevention." *Clinical Pediatrics*, 1966, *5*, 187-190.

The Use of Crisis Intervention

AUTHOR: A. L. Rosenkrantz

PRECIS: Understanding suicidal behavior as a crisis reaction in a chronically stressed individual and providing both crisis intervention and long-term therapy

INTRODUCTION: Recent statistics indicate a suicide rate of twelve per hundred thousand in the United States. A disproportionate number of suicides are committed by persons in the fifteen to twenty-four age group, and there is a trend toward increasing numbers of suicides among this group. Rosenkrantz reports on research stressing the importance of problems with self-identity and intimacy in the etiology of suicidal behavior. He particularly emphasizes confusion in sexual identity and notes the contribution of family breakup and lack of clarity in societal definitions of sex roles to sexual identity problems. He also comments on the role of parental rejection in precipitating suicide and points out that the most significant precipitating event for suicide is the loss through death, desertion, or separation of some important person.

TREATMENT METHOD: Crisis intervention techniques are seen as particularly appropriate for suicidal adolescents. Clients can be encouraged to enter into a "no suicide contract" while the precipitating events are explored further. The therapist works at bringing out the client's ambivalence regarding suicide while conveying his or her understanding and acceptance of the feelings that led to this behavior. As the therapist works to alleviate the precipitating crisis, he or she should also seek to build a therapeutic alliance that can support further exploration of more chronic problems.

When the precipitating event is a loss the client has not been able to accept, Rosenkrantz suggests using a Gestalt therapy technique called the "two chair method" to work through conflicting feelings. The client alternates between being himself or herself and playing the part of the lost love object. A dialogue that permits feelings to be expressed is established. Through this exercise the client is able to express his or her anger and sadness regarding the loss and to arrive at some acceptable way of saying goodbye to the departed person.

Regarding the issue of assessing the potential for further suicidal behavior, Rosenkrantz, following J. P. Wollersheem ("The Assessment of Suicide Potential by Interview Methods," *Psychotherapy, Research and Practice*, 1974, *11*, 222-225), suggests exploring such things as the frequency of suicidal ideation, explicitness of planning, and the client's capacity for self-control.

COMMENTARY: Rosenkrantz provides a general framework for carrying out psychotherapy with a suicidal adolescent and suggests specific techniques for dealing with the immediate crisis. He does not go into detail regarding techniques for working on long-term, chronic problems. He makes suggestions regarding the assessment of suicidal risk, but he does not go far enough in this regard. One should also be concerned about mental status when assessing suicide risk, particularly if there is evidence of depression or thought disturbance and if the client reports that voices are telling him to kill himself. Understanding of family dynamics and intrafamily stresses is important in assessing risk as well as in planning treatment. When there has already been one suicide attempt, the client's reaction to failure is also an important factor to consider.

SOURCE: Rosenkrantz, A. L. "A Note on Adolescent Suicide: Incidence, Dynamics, and Some Suggestions for Treatment." *Adolescence*, 1978, *13*, 209-214.

The Use of Insight Therapy

AUTHORS: A. Shrut and T. Michels

PRECIS: Long-term management of the suicidal adolescent with emphasis on understanding unconscious motivations

INTRODUCTION: Shrut and Michels report on the treatment of a group of fourteen female adolescents who attempted suicide. The most frequently used method was drug ingestion. Most of the girls came from unstable families, and there was typically a history of strife between the two parents and between at least one of the parents and the child. These girls saw themselves as rejected and had in many cases gotten the message from their parents that things really would be better if they weren't around. For some, rejection by a boyfriend or a lover precipitated the suicide attempt; but even so, this usually recapitulated a pattern that had been established in the home. The authors describe their approach to treatment for these girls and present specific case examples.

CASE HISTORY: Miss N. was a thirteen-year-old girl who lived with her divorced mother. An argument between mother and daughter about the daughter's household responsibilities precipitated the attempt. Initial assessment suggested that several motivations were operating: a desire to get away from the mother, to force her to be more concerned, and to punish her for her lack of caring. The patient was obviously ambivalent about her suicide and showed a strong will to live. Therapy was conducted almost exclusively through family interviews. Mother and daughter learned to understand and empathize with each other as the therapist encouraged each to talk about personal concerns in the presence of the other. The daughter learned of her mother's difficulties as a single working parent, and the mother became aware of her daughter's feelings that neither of her parents really cared for her.

Miss C. was a young woman of nineteen who took an overdose of pills and stabbed herself in the abdomen after her boyfriend rejected her. She indicated that she wanted to make him suffer. She stated, "I'm not dirty, and he'll know he loved me when I'm dead." Therapy focused primarily on helping this girl to understand how unconscious motivations adversely influenced her relationships with other people. Salient motivational and behavior patterns included a need to undo a rejecting home life by forcing men to love her, repetitively setting up rejections, a tendency to pursue men who rejected her and reject men who pursued her, and guilt feelings about attaining a sexual relationship with any man. A major task for therapy was to alert the client to how old habits and attitudes toward her parents influenced her relationships with other people in the present. The goal was to develop self-awareness so that she recognized when she was falling into a self-defeating habit and change her behavior accordingly.

TREATMENT METHOD: The major concern initially is the establishment of a strong therapeutic alliance. To facilitate this, Shrut and Michels recommend seeing the adolescent first and hearing her side of the story before talking to other family members and also seeing her again at the close of the initial session. The therapist must quickly make a decision about the risk of further attempts, and often a brief period of hospitalization is necessary to make certain that background history and precipitating events are understood and that the situation is under control. Therapy involves environmental manipulation as well as insight-oriented interviews. A family focus is necessary, even when family members are not seen as a group. In individual therapy, the client is helped to see how parents have exerted a destructive influence on his or her life, but as the treatment bond becomes stronger, clients are increasingly encouraged to take responsibility for their own attitudes and actions. Shrut and Michels feel that a major obstacle to successful treatment is the client's unwillingness to give up immature desires for excessive power and importance.

COMMENTARY: The cases presented range from one involving a relatively simple application of family counseling to overcome

a child's concerns about acceptance to a very complicated case
in which destructive parents had led a young woman to virtual
despair of ever being accepted. The two cases together point up
the need for a flexible approach that uses a variety of treatment
techniques, depending on such factors as severity of problem,
availability for treatment of key family members, and age and
developmental stage of the client. For the second case presented, even greater flexibility of treatment approach might
have been beneficial. Systematic desensitization, for example,
could have been utilized to reduce anxieties about sexuality,
and at least some irrational beliefs could probably have been attacked directly without exploring their unconscious sources. A
systematic approach to self-reinforcement for appropriate social
behavior could have been used in overcoming self-defeating behaviors in interpersonal relationships.

SOURCE: Shrut, A., and Michels, T. "Adolescent Girls Who
    Attempt Suicide—Comments on Treatment." *American Jour-
    nal of Psychotherapy,* 1969, *23,* 243-251.

Treatment Issues with Suicidal
Adolescents

AUTHOR: J. A. Motto

PRECIS: Special considerations in the treatment of suicidal
adolescents and their families

INTRODUCTION: Many of the factors that make adolescents
difficult to treat are especially problematic in the treatment of
suicidal adolescents. Their "now" orientation coupled with the
tendency to communicate through action rather than words increase the risk of impulsive suicidal behavior. Ambivalence about
dependency and fear of rejection both work against establish-

ment of the interpersonal trust that is so important in reducing suicide potential.

TREATMENT METHOD: Motto describes the initial work with the suicidal adolescent as a mixture of both assessment and treatment. A prime objective is the establishment of a dependent relationship that will support further therapeutic work. This initial treatment goal can be achieved at the same time assessment is being carried out if the therapist is an empathic listener who communicates respect and avoids passing judgment on the client's behavior. Motto urges using an indirect approach in assessing motivating factors for the suicide. He feels that direct questioning of why the attempt was made is often perceived as accusatory and that in the process of eliciting information about school, social life, and family, the therapist can usually clarify the origins of the self-destructive impulse. Once the client develops a sense of being able to depend upon the therapist for emotional gratification, the therapist can begin to make demands for therapeutic work. The focus should be on overcoming the unique stresses being experienced by this particular client. These often include such things as anxieties about sexual identity, anger toward parents, and low self-esteem. The family should be involved in both assessment and treatment. Contact with other family members can help clarify motivations for the suicide; they can assist with removing possible instruments of suicide from the home environment; and they can be involved in efforts to change their own behaviors that may be directly related to the client's low self-esteem and feelings of despair.

SPECIAL CONSIDERATIONS: Motto lists a number of specific guidelines in the treatment of suicidal adolescents:

1. Use an inpatient treatment setting until it is clear that the continued risk of suicide is minimal. When handled properly, hospitalization gives a clear message that a cry for help has been heard and is being taken seriously.
2. Be cautious in accepting the client's reassurances that he or she will not make further suicide attempts.

3. If treatment is to be done on an outpatient basis, make certain that appointments are scheduled without delay. Continue with the therapist who managed the initial crisis if at all possible.

4. Be flexible about scheduling, especially in the beginning, even if it means allowing the client to be somewhat manipulative.

5. Avoid glib reassurances, which may communicate a lack of understanding of the seriousness of the adolescent's predicament.

6. Avoid casual banter, which may be misinterpreted as disapproval or rejection.

7. Foster a variety of relationships in addition to the therapeutic alliance.

8. Emphasize stability in relationships by discouraging prolonged absences of people to whom the client is attached.

9. Be prepared for a stormy course of therapy. It is easy for the therapist to become defensive or even hostile toward such a client.

10. Arrange for a colleague to act as a backup consultant. In the event that a crisis develops in the therapeutic relationship, do not hesitate to use this resource.

Discharge from the hospital, reduced frequency of sessions, therapist vacations, and movement toward termination are all critical points in the treatment that require careful preparation. Adequate preparations include advance discussion regarding impending changes, reassurance regarding continued interest and availability, development of alternative supportive relationships, and provision for follow-up appointments.

The therapist should be prepared for the possibility that, despite his or her efforts, a suicide may occur. It then becomes a part of the therapist's responsibility to follow through with family members, helping them deal with their anger, guilt, and feelings of personal loss.

COMMENTARY: Motto describes assessment and treatment with suicidal adolescents and provides specific guidelines for managing the therapeutic relationship. He points out the value of using an indirect approach in assessing suicidal motivation and emphasizes the need for building a strong therapeutic alliance to support subsequent therapeutic work. Although using an indirect approach is probably beneficial in promoting the therapeutic relationship, there are times when direct questioning is also needed. The therapist must certainly engage in some fairly direct questioning about suicidal ideation and suicidal plans; and, as Bratter (see Additional Readings) points out, there are times when a direct approach may be a prerequisite to the establishment of a working alliance. The specific guidelines Motto provides for managing the therapeutic relationship are thorough and should be useful to any therapist involved in adolescent treatment.

SOURCE: Motto, J. A. "Treatment and Management of Suicidal Adolescents." *Psychiatric Opinion,* 1975, *12,* 14-20.

Family Crisis Intervention

AUTHORS: G. C. Morrison and J. G. Collier

PRECIS: Family crisis intervention in the treatment of the suicidal adolescent

INTRODUCTION: Suicide attempts almost invariably reflect acute emotional distress. Morrison and Collier believe that the distress of the suicidal adolescent stems as much from disturbance in family function as from individual problems, and they view the crisis of a suicide attempt as an opportunity to effect a family change that will decrease the likelihood of such behavior in the future.

Thirty-four families were provided with crisis intervention treatment after a child made a suicide attempt or serious threat.

Sixty-five percent of these young people were between the ages of fifteen and seventeen, and most of them were girls. A variety of symptoms was present in addition to the suicidal behavior, including school refusal, truancy, sexual promiscuity, hyperactivity, social withdrawal, assaultiveness, running away, and drug or alcohol use. In approximately 75 percent of the cases, the family had experienced a significant loss or separation or the anniversary of such in the weeks preceding the suicide attempt.

CASE HISTORY: The case of the Brown family is illustrative of case material presented. They came for emergency treatment after their seventeen-year-old daughter, Sharon, attempted suicide. Sharon was a high school senior whose mother had been hospitalized because of acute depression. Though she had been awarded a college scholarship, Sharon dropped out of high school, apparently in response to excessive demands placed on her by her family. Father and sister seemed unable to cope with the prospect of doing without both Sharon and her mother if she went away to college. After much ventilation of feeling, the problem was defined as one of anxiety on the part of all family members about separation and about changing accustomed patterns of living. The clinical team played down the separation aspects of Sharon's going to college, indicating that there would be frequent opportunities for visiting; and the threat to family stability was reduced by mother's return from the hospital. Sharon did go to college and was still enrolled at one-year follow-up.

TREATMENT METHOD: Treatment was provided by a team consisting of child psychiatrist and social worker. The initial step was a "diagnostic-therapeutic" interview involving all significant family members. The interview was directed toward identifying particular stresses that had precipitated the suicide attempt as well as family dynamics that had led to vulnerability to these stresses. The goal was to arrive at a definition of problems that was acceptable to family members and to clinical staff. The team then saw the family for as long as necessary to resolve the crisis (usually three or four interviews).

TREATMENT RESULTS: Some families were able to develop communication skills that could be used in solving other problems, and some families were unable to get beyond resolving the immediate crisis. In most cases, referrals were made for follow-up treatment, but compliance was generally poor once the crisis was over.

COMMENTARY: Treatment for suicidal adolescents and their families is usually described as involving two stages, crisis intervention and follow-up treatment. Although the latter is almost always indicated, many families fail to follow through once the suicidal crisis has been alleviated. For these families, access to the crisis unit and preferably to a particular team within that unit should be kept open. Long-term goals formulated in time of crisis can then be integrated with subsequent crisis interventions.

SOURCE: Morrison, G. C., and Collier, J. G. "Family Treatment Approaches to Suicidal Children and Adolescents." *Journal of the American Academy of Child Psychiatry,* 1969, *8,* 140-153.

Treating the Families of Suicidal Adolescents

AUTHOR: M. Kerfoot

PRECIS: Reassigning family tasks to relieve the pressures of role reversal

INTRODUCTION: The importance of family dynamics in the etiology of suicidal behavior is often stressed. Kerfoot describes a specific dynamic, role reversal, that has been manifest in the families of many of the suicidal adolescents whom he has treated. In role reversal, parents display helplessness and dependency and the child displays a reciprocal nuturing and caretaking behavior appropriate to the parental role. This reversal is initiated by the parent, and generally the child feels unable to resist it. Kerfoot feels that adolescents are particularly vulnerable to such pressure because differences between child and parent are less clear at this point in development and because readiness to experiment with new roles is a normal part of adolescence.

The adolescent who is caught in a role reversal situation has his or her freedom seriously curtailed at a time when having freedom is particularly important to development. Frustration and anger are the natural result. Low self-esteem stemming from inadequacies in carrying out role demands is also present and is often exacerbated by parental criticism. Conflicting peer pressures add to the adolescent's sense of frustration. For some, a suicidal attempt offers a temporary way out that also restores them to a dependent position.

CASE HISTORY: Janet was a fifteen-year-old girl living with her parents and a younger brother. Mother's physical and emotional health had deteriorated due to illness and heavy drinking. Father worked nights and had minimal contact with his wife. As mother became less capable, Janet assumed various parental functions, including that of making sure her mother got off to work on time. When Janet's boyfriend began making additional demands on her time, she was placed in a difficult dilemma. A dispute with her mother ultimately precipitated a suicide attempt through drug ingestion.

Tracy was an eleven-year-old girl who had been pressed into assuming parental duties at the age of six, when her mother gave birth to an unplanned and unwanted child. Her mother became extremely depressed and increasingly unable to function, and her father was unable to take up the slack because of a serious alcohol problem. Tracy had difficulty concentrating on the normal pursuits of a school-age girl because of her excessive emotional involvement with her mother, and ultimately her school performance began to deteriorate. When the stresses fi-

nally became too much for her, she made a suicide attempt
through drug ingestion.

TREATMENT METHOD: Treatment in the first case involved
restructuring the family so that family members could assume
their appropriate roles. Janet's mother was referred to an alcoholism treatment unit, and Janet was given emotional support
to continue in a semiparental role during the early stages of her
mother's treatment. Janet's father was helped to understand his
daughter's developmental needs and encouraged to become a
more active parent who could provide her with practical and
emotional support in her difficult relationship with her mother.

Treatment in the second case again involved restructuring
the family by promoting behaviors appropriate to each member's family role. This time the father was referred for treatment of alcoholism, and the mother was involved in therapy sessions. The therapist temporarily assumed some of the parental
decision-making responsibilities while helping mother to master
the skills necessary for this role. Tracy was involved in a therapy group in which she could work on social skills deficiencies
that prevented her from entering into normal peer relationships.

COMMENTARY: Kerfoot has found a logical point of entry
into the multiproblem families of his suicidal adolescent patients. Obviously, role reversal is not the only problem or even
the most serious problem for these families, but it does provide
a focus for treatment. The restructuring that the therapist carries out is at times a compromise between the possible and the
ideal. In the first case, for example, there was no one who could
assume all the parental functions the mother had relinquished
to her daughter, and the daughter was left with some of these
even after the problem was recognized. With respect to the second case, it should be noted that recognizing the problem and
restructuring the family cannot undo years of deprivation in experience with normal developmental tasks. Therapy often requires compensating for these missed opportunities, as was done
for this girl in her group therapy experience.

SOURCE: Kerfoot, M. "Parent-Child Role Reversal and Adolescent Suicidal Behavior." *Journal of Adolescence,* 1979, 2, 337-343.

Cognitive Approaches in the Treatment of Suicide

AUTHOR: K. Glaser

PRECIS: Cognitive approaches to alleviating depression for adolescents who attempt suicide

INTRODUCTION: Loss and abandonment play an important role in the etiology of adolescent depression and suicidal behavior. Loss of self-esteem is also a major factor. Glaser points out that adolescents are particularly vulnerable to distortions in self-concept, which aggravate self-esteem problems. These distortions include unrealistic self-expectations and a tendency to interpret single instances of success or failure as valid indicators of self-worth. He notes that concerns about loss and abandonment are particularly salient among adopted children and children in foster care and that low self-esteem is often a problem for the neurologically impaired child and children with learning handicaps.

TREATMENT METHOD: Glaser recommends an active approach to the treatment of depressed and suicidal adolescents. This involves assisting directly in removing obstacles to important goals, providing direct advice, and consulting directly with parents, teachers, and others who are importantly involved in the clients well-being. He places special emphasis on promoting realistic self-appraisal. This can be fostered by exercises that require clients to rate themselves on a variety of dimensions in relation to an appropriate reference group. Global dimensions like intelligence can be broken down into specific component skills. School achievement can be broken into specific subjects, and physical and personality attributes can also be considered. Clients should be helped to see themselves as having many dimensions and having strengths in some areas that balance perceived weaknesses in others. In addition, clients are helped to distinguish between alterable and unalterable characteristics and given direct assistance in achieving change where change is desired. The therapist takes an active role in directing the client into activities where success is likely, for example, a particular recreational activity, special school, or vocational training program. Environmental manipulations like changing a child to a class that provides a more favorable reference group can also be considered. Parents are counseled regarding realistic levels of expectation and urged to set their sights in such a way that success is likely.

Glaser emphasizes that there are risks as well as benefits in the hospitalization of suicidal adolescents. He points out that hospitalization can be seen as rejection or abandonment and that resulting anger can increase motivation to retaliate through suicidal behavior. He suggests a number of factors that should be considered in the decision for hospitalization. These include pervasiveness of current stresses, degree of impulse control, availability of an adequate support system outside the treatment setting, and the therapist's willingness and ability to involve himself or herself in crisis management outside the treatment hour.

COMMENTARY: Glaser makes a valuable contribution by highlighting the cognitive factors in depression. People do become depressed and even suicidal when they evaluate themselves negatively, and the frame of reference for these evaluations can be quite arbitrary. One can influence self-evaluation by helping the client to adopt a different reference group or by actually making changes in the groups to which he or she belongs. As has been noted in the chapter on emotional disorders, one can also alleviate depression by encouraging selective remembrance of specific facts or experiences. Finally, there is the possibility of actually changing one's position on some dimensions, especially if a therapist takes an active role in supporting such changes.

SOURCE: Glaser, K. "The Treatment of Depressed and Suicidal Adolescents." *American Journal of Psychotherapy*, 1978, *32*, 252-269.

Desensitization in the Treatment of Suicide

AUTHORS: T. Elliott, R. Smith, and R. Wildman

PRECIS: Reducing suicidal behavior by decreasing suicidal thoughts and by applying desensitization to anxiety-arousing thoughts that precipitate suicidal behavior

INTRODUCTION: For clients who repeatedly attempt suicide, the thoughts and feelings that usually precipitate an attempt can be elicited and specific training can be introduced to reduce their impact. Suicidal thinking can also be paired with an unpleasant sensation, reducing the likelihood of both suicidal thoughts and behaviors.

CASE HISTORY: The client was a fourteen-year-old girl who had repeatedly attempted suicide by slashing her wrists. She came from a very unsatisfactory home environment, and by age seven had already been placed with a foster care agency. Subsequently, she was placed in a juvenile detention center and then in the psychiatric hospital where she resided at the time of treatment. Her suicide attempts generally occurred when she was angry or upset and when she began thinking about her past.

TREATMENT METHOD: Treatment was carried out in two phases. The first was directed toward decreasing suicidal thinking. The client was taught how to control muscle tension and relaxation and then taught to relax when looking at a picture of herself socializing with a friend and to tense when looking at a picture of herself applying a piece of broken glass to her wrist. Later she was taught to tense and relax appropriately while imagining such situations and to do so without prompting by her therapist. For the second phase, a list of anxiety-generating thoughts that typically led to suicidal behavior was constructed. These were arranged in a hierarchy from least to most anxiety provoking. Using the relaxation skills she had already acquired, the client was taught to relax while imagining each item in the hierarchy, starting with the least anxiety arousing and working progressively toward the item that evoked the greatest anxiety. These ranged from thoughts of not living at home with her family to the high anxiety item of handling sharp objects.

TREATMENT RESULTS: Suicidal attempts were reduced from an average of 3 to .17 per month. There were no attempts during the last seven months of follow up.

COMMENTARY: A modified desensitization approach was highly successful for this client. The application of this method does, however, seem to depend on a history of multiple attempts using the same method. The first phase of treatment would certainly have been much more complicated if all attempts had not been made by wrist slashing, and the second phase required finding a pattern in precipitating thoughts and images over multiple attempts. In some cases it might be advantageous to use shock or some other aversive stimulus in place of tension training in the first phase of treatment, although using tension and relaxation together does have the advantage of simultaneously weakening the target behavior and promoting a desirable alternative.

SOURCE: Elliott, T., Smith, D., and Wildman, R. "Suicide and Systematic Desensitization: A Case Study." *Journal of Clinical Psychology,* 1972, *28,* 420-423.

Additional Readings

Bratter, T. E. "Responsible Therapeutic Eros: The Psychotherapist Who Cares Enough to Define and Enforce Behavior Limits with Potentially Suicidal Adolescents." *Counseling Psychologist,* 1975, *5,* 97-104.

Bratter describes his work with self-destructive adolescent drug abusers and the problems involved in treating them. He states that their anger, defiance, attempts to intimidate, and reluctance to get involved all preclude traditional approaches to therapy. He argues that, at least initially, the basic issue is survival and that the therapist must take an authoritarian stance to contain suicidal behavior. He sees this limit setting as essential to the establishment of a therapeutic alliance and argues that it is only after the therapist has demonstrated that he or she cares enough to take control that the client becomes available for other therapeutic work.

Greuling, J. W., and De Blassic, R. R. "Adolescent Suicide." *Adolescence,* 1980, *15,* 589-601.

The authors review research findings on adolescent suicide and make recommendations regarding prevention and treatment. They indicate that school counselors are in a good position both to detect individuals at risk and to carry out prevention programs. They argue that nondirective counseling for those in the at-risk group should be effective in decreasing the incidence of suicide attempts. Recommendations for treatment of those who actually make attempts include family crisis intervention and individual and family therapy. Signposts of long-term progress are suggested. These include improvements in self-concept, family and peer relationships, and academic functioning, as well as increased interest in outside activity and decreases in other psychiatric symptomatology.

Hochberg, R. "Psychotherapy of a Suicidal Boy: Dynamics and Interventions." *Psychotherapy: Theory, Research, and Practice,* 1977, *14,* 428-433.

Hochberg reports on the successful treatment of a seventeen-year-old boy who attempted suicide by drug ingestion. Rejection by his peers and loneliness were his stated reasons for the suicide attempt, though it subsequently emerged that his reaction to a homosexual experience was also an important factor. Treatment was initially carried out on an outpatient basis, but a period of hospitalization was necessary when the patient indicated that he could no longer keep a "no suicide contract." Hospital treatment included individual, group, and family therapies, all of which contributed to the ultimate positive outcome. The patient gradually gained confidence in taking a more masculine role and in being more self-sufficient. Treatment was successfully terminated at the time of his going away to college.

Kerfoot, M. "The Family Context of Adolescent Suicidal Behavior." *Journal of Adolescence,* 1980, *3,* 335-346.

Kerfoot describes family and psychodynamic factors associated with adolescent suicide and points out the need to take the family into account in treatment planning. Specific problems requiring attention include disharmony between the parents, poor communication within the family, and parental indifference to or outright rejection of their child. High expectations and excessive control are also seen as elements in the family context of suicidal adolescents. The young person living in such a family feels unworthy, rejected, and helpless. Having no outlet for resulting feelings of rage, he turns them inward in self-destructive behavior.

McAnarney, E. R. "Adolescent and Young Adult Suicide in the United States—A Reflection of Societal Unrest." *Adolescence,* 1979, *14,* 765-774.

Adolescent and young adult suicides in the United States have been increasing over the past twenty years. McAnarney has reviewed the literature on suicide to discover factors that might be responsible for this increase. Family factors seem particularly important. Where family ties are strong, suicide rates are low. Many suicide attempters come from broken homes or homes in which they have experienced a succession of caretakers. Suicide rates are high in transient or mobile groups and particularly among immigrant populations. Suicide rates are also high in groups in which direct expression of angry feelings is suppressed.

Pfeffer, C. R. "Suicidal Behavior of Children: A Review with
Implications for Research and Practice." *American Journal of
Psychiatry*, 1981, *138*, 154-159.

Pfeffer provides a thorough review of the literature on suicide among children in the six- to twelve-year age range. She
notes that, although the incidence of completed suicides is quite
low during these years, suicide threats and attempts occur more
frequently. These can be viewed as early warnings of greater suicide risk in adolescence. Pfeffer emphasizes the supportive role
of teachers, clergy, police, and others who work directly in the
community in the identification of potentially suicidal children
and notes that their ability to function effectively is enhanced
when the psychiatrist is available as a consultant. Psychiatrists
are urged to consider suicide risk for all children referred for
psychiatric evaluation, regardless of the referral problem.

Wenz, F. "Sociological Correlates of Alienation Among Adolescent Suicide Attempts." *Adolescence*, 1979, *14*, 19-30.

A relationship has been hypothesized between suicide in
adolescence and alienation. Wenz defines alienation as meaning
"not regulated by society" and "not able to influence society."
Using a twenty-item scale to measure this variable, he assessed
correlations between alienation and other variables thought to
be related to suicide potential. The subjects for his study were
two hundred suicide attempters. Within this group, degree of
alienation correlated positively with coming from a broken
home, having communication problems with parents, being in
conflict with parents, having step-parents, and having experienced a broken romance. There were negative correlations with
amount of social contact with peers, economic status of parents, and school performance.

Yusin, A. S. "Attempted Suicide in an Adolescent—The Resolution of an Anxiety State." *Adolescence*, 1973, *8*, 17-28.

Yusin reports on the case of a sixteen-year-old girl, Martha,
who attempted suicide by cutting her wrists and drinking rub-
bing alcohol. Throughout the first six years of her life, Martha
experienced chronic fighting between her parents and frequent
neglect by her mother. At age six, she was raped by an older

cousin, and she was made to feel that this was her fault. In the same year, her parents separated, though they did not actually get divorced until she was thirteen (a divorce that she was unable to accept). At the time of the divorce, she began withdrawing from peer relationships, apparently because her friends were critical of her relationships with boys. She had many boyfriends but each time terminated the relationship when the boys became interested in her sexually. The precipitating event for the suicide attempt was her breakup with a boyfriend after she refused his sexual advances. Yusin saw her as using sexual attractiveness to meet dependency needs without real awareness that it stimulated sexual desire. Suicide was seen as a means of coping with intolerable feelings that she was alone and abandoned and that something horrible was about to happen.

Author Index

Subject Index

A

Abuse, and lack of assertiveness, 173-174

Acting out: characteristics of, 212; controls for, 216-218; family therapy for, 221-222, 224; genesis of, 223; interventions for, 212-224; involuntary treatment for, 216-218; limit setting for, 214; and paraprofessionals, 216, 217; psychoanalytic approach to, 213-215; rational behavior therapy for, 218-220; readings on, 223-224; relaxation for, 223; support and uncovering for, 217; therapy for, 223-224

Adolescents: antisocial behavior by, 187-263; developmental tasks of, 1-2, 59-60, 71-73, 265; emotional disorders of, 11-61; fear in, of being defective, 4; impulsive, and delinquency, 249-251, 257-259; impulsive, and running away, 195-197; and independence, struggle for, 6; interpersonal skills deficits of, 133-185; period of, 1; physical disorders of, 63-132; separation of, from family discord, 138-140; sexual